D1583010

Problems and Solutions
in Complete Denture Prosthodontics

David J. Lamb

Quintessence Publishing Co., Inc. 1993
London, Chicago, Berlin, São Paulo and Tokyo

First published 1993 by
Quintessence Publishing Company Ltd
London, UK

© 1993 Quintessence Publishing Co. Ltd

ISBN 1-85097-021-1

Printed and bound in Great Britain by
Biddles Ltd, Guildford and King's Lynn
from typesetting by AsTec, Saffron Walden

Contents

Foreword

This book sets out in an imaginative way to interest, educate and instruct all those who are treating edentulousness and admirably achieves these aims.

It has to be recognised that the successful treatment of patients requiring complete dentures is becoming more difficult for the patient, the dental surgeon and the technician. There is a need for the practitioner to have a thorough grasp of methods of patient assessment as well as knowledge of good basic prosthetic techniques. In addition, there is the requirement for the dental team to have both adequate time to treat and a wide knowledge of all the various special techniques that may be utilised to benefit patients. Every patient requires an individual, specialised approach and, as we move forward to treating the increasingly difficult clinical condition of edentulousness in an ageing population in the 21st century, all of their skills will be required.

Textbooks on prosthetic dentistry so often involve a detailed description of didactic approaches to the subject and this can be very unsatisfactory for those with a deep existing interest in, and an adequate knowledge of, the subject. This book overcomes that difficulty by assuming that readers will have these attributes.

Because this book has a practical, sensible approach with a wealth of information for us to help our patients, it will, I am sure, be widely useful for practitioners and students of all ages.

Derek Stafford MSc, PhD, FDSRCS
Professor of Prosthetic Dentistry
University of Wales
College of Medicine

Preface

Readers may be surprised to find that although the text is arranged in normal clinical sequence for one on complete dentures, they may not find in the various sections details of their normal impression technique or their favourite system of registering the jaw relations. This book is not designed to teach basic complete denture prosthodontics. The students and practitioners for whom it is written will already have acquired basic clinical skills, and their bookshelves will already be well stocked with appropriate texts. Their need is for an encapsulation and analysis of the difficulties inherent in this discipline and a summary of the best approach to a satisfactory solution for their patients' problems. The problems discussed are those likely to be encountered in practice by a general dental practitioner. To this end it concerns itself with practical techniques and their application. It is not intended to be a text for the specialist in maxillo-facial prosthetics or the dental implantologist. Where I have enlarged on some aspect of a related discipline it is because I have felt it to be within the scope of the interested practitioner without extensive additional training.

References flourish in scientific articles where even the most common knowledge appears to demand the support of multiple citations. Whether or not there should be references in a clinical textbook can be debated. A book may take a year to bring from final draft to publication, and any references in it are either out of date or common knowledge almost from the time of printing. For this reason opinions differ whether extensive citation of references serves a valid purpose.

References nevertheless perform a useful function and permit serious readers to increase their understanding of ideas that are of interest. When the "name and date" system of citation was popular the text was disrupted by their inclusion. Today, systems involving superscript numbers are almost universal and citations can be included without causing an interruption in continuity. I have therefore included a number of references which enlarge further on processes and techniques and at least serve as a jumping-off point to the literature. I have taken care to select those that are recent (the majority are from the last 10 years) and are easily accessible in most libraries. Any not fulfilling these criteria are included because of their importance. I have cited few textbooks, not because I consider their contents unimportant, but because the ideas they incorporate are so important that they will be already well known to the reader.

I apologise for any repetition. Inevitably techniques and ideas have repeated themselves in some of the chapters. To avoid excessive use of the phrase "see chapter . . ." and the search this involves, I have at times allowed myself the luxury of a summary of the relevant work.

DJL
April, 1992

Acknowledgements

I would like to thank Professor R. B. Johns for permission to reproduce Figs. 1.18, 1.20 and 8.3, and Mr I. M. Brook for allowing me to use Fig. 1.5. Ultimately any prosthodontist is at the mercy of his technicians, and my thanks go especially to the technical staff of the Department of Restorative Dentistry at Sheffield, for their good natured help and support at all times.

Chapter 1

Patient Assessment

A recent study has shown that losing teeth and having complete dentures made is a stressful event comparable in significance to marriage, retirement and changing careers.[1] For patients unfortunate enough to lose all their teeth, the importance of comfortable, efficient complete dentures cannot be overemphasized. Their contribution to quality of life is considerable and they allow better adjustment to life's problems. Frequently the practitioner's road to patient satisfaction is signposted by a succession of problems and necessitates detours round unsuperable obstacles, but because the importance of the end product is so great the extra effort gives great professional pleasure.

Many of the problems encountered in complete denture prosthodontics can be avoided by careful assessment. It is always tempting to neglect this stage and think that treatment is simplified by loss of the teeth. Once the patient is in the surgery, it is then assumed that any problems can be dealt with as they are encountered. This is never the correct course, and after taking care to ensure good communication with the patient, a careful history and examination are essential.

Communication

The first need in assessment is good communication and an understanding of patient behaviour. In dental schools formal student training is mainly directed to the acquisition of clinical and technical skills plus the background of physical and biological sciences necessary for their successful application. It is provided and supervised by staff whose career progress is determined in part by their clinical and teaching expertise but principally by their ability at scientific research and scholarship. The natural sciences tend, therefore, to be emphasized at the expense of the social and behavioural sciences. Much of a student's interpersonal skill and understanding of patients' motives is picked up unconsciously and in an unstructured way through the hidden curriculum which is provided by interaction with staff of all grades, in the day-to-day treatment of patients, and in the normal social round. Only recently has communication entered the curriculum as a subject in its own right, and most of a practitioner's communication skills will continue to be picked up piecemeal following graduation.

9

It is difficult to understand why so little emphasis is placed on this aspect of behavioural science. In purely financial terms communication skills are of obvious benefit. It has been estimated that over a 5-year period about 25% of patients are lost as a result of poor dentist/patient communication.[2] There are also other financial advantages. It is known that best results are achieved when treating a co-operative, informed patient, and the creation of a satisfactory dentist/patient relationship has a powerful therapeutic effect. When communication is good, patients comply better with instructions and, equally importantly, the amount of information provided by a relaxed, interested patient promotes greater understanding of any problem.

The obstacles to communication tend to be mostly on the dentist's side as he tries to maintain control of the "interview". The attitude of domination is appealing as it feeds the need to be a person of decision and action. But while it satisfies the clinician's ego and cuts down on time-wasting digressions, it does so by restricting the flow of information. The other apparent advantage of a dominating attitude is that it decreases uncertainty in the mind of both the dentist and the patient. This might be an advantage in those disciplines where treatment and success are clear cut, but in complete denture prosthodontics, where success can be partial or relative, a patient's initial certainty that treatment will be successful can end in disenchantment unless their expectations are tempered by the understanding which follows adequate communication.

How to improve communication

Good verbal communication is a habit which becomes a reflex with practice. It is a habit which is made easier to acquire by interest in our profession, our professional abilities, and our patients. Once the importance of communication is emphasized, the necessary skills are merely common sense and quickly applied. There are, however, a few ways in which the process can be made easier.

It is accepted that the dental surgery is not the ideal place for friendly conversation; even the word clinical, which means "at the bedside", has overtones of sterility, sharpness, efficiency and patient vulnerability. Even to an edentulous patient the surgery is strange and full of unknown hazards. The clothes of the dentist and his assistant are often formal and off-putting. As a first stage, therefore, seat the patient at their ease, and, sitting opposite, attempt to overcome by word and manner the impediments to free communication.

As dentists we are fairly typical members of our socio-economic group, and tend to assume that most patients have a level of intelligence and social skills approaching our own. Sometimes we even expect from our patients the same degree of interest in things dental. In communication with some patients our very obvious social advantages can have an inhibiting effect. We must be prepared for this and, without appearing to patronize, be ready to spend adequate time, even giving the extra instructions and information we are *not* asked for. Also, importantly, we have to remember that a patient's lack of status does not imply that their interest in dental care has an equally low priority.

Related to this is that other stumbling block, the use of jargon. When dealing with fellow professionals, jargon is necessary for the sake of accuracy, but with patients it acts as a barrier. No one likes to admit to ignorance, but unwillingness to ask the meaning of a jargon word might prevent important details being provided and stifle the free flow of information. It can even prevent the understanding of instructions and be instrumental in causing the high degree of non-compliance which characterizes the patient response to professional advice.[3]

Many complete denture patients are elderly and special problems are encountered in communication. Deafness is common and requires tact and careful management to avoid giving offence. High-frequency hearing is the first to be lost. Parts of words will be misunderstood and in the resulting confusion we may compensate by shouting. This merely embarrasses the patient, and loud shouting can cause physical pain. Speak slowly and clearly for maximum comprehension. The worst barrier is a tendency to believe that the elderly are less intellectually competent than "normal" mature adults. By giving a childish, over-simplistic explanation it is easy to create negative attitudes and a communication barrier.

All problems with communication can be solved by understanding and time, but clinical time is at a premium. Patients' time, too, is valuable and we can help with a little forethought and refinement of our questioning skills. Remember, we start off with the advantage that most patients have initial good will towards us. When in due course we ask, "What is the problem with your dentures?", and receive the apparently uninformative reply, "Well, they all say that my upper gum has shrunk", followed by comments on the inferior abilities of previous dentists—which it seems impolite to interrupt—take it not as a digression but as a complement. The patient has answered the question not by reference to the problem that *they* have but by the problem *you* will have, and have given a sure sign of their good intentions and willingness to help. If this is thought to waste too much time, then perhaps at the next opportunity if the question is rephrased as "What is the problem which makes you think your dentures need to be replaced?", we might get, "Because my upper denture tips down at the back when I bite on my front teeth", or other equally brief and helpful reply.

History

Personal details

One of the effects of the present emphasis on preventive dentistry and the improvements in general health and clinical dental techniques that have come about over the last few decades, is that edentulous patients form a smaller but increasingly elderly group, and with greater longevity have to wear complete dentures to an advanced age. With the passage of time all people gradually lose their ability to adapt to new circumstances. Hence, of the personal details by far the most important is the patient's chronological age, although this must be modified by an assessment of the patient's physiological age and the extent to which they interact positively with their environment. The prognosis for an interested, mentally active 70-year-old must always be better than that for a lethargic, inward-looking 60-year-old.

Where a satisfactory set of complete dentures has been worn for some years by an elderly patient, with the gradual deterioration in fit that we would expect, satisfaction is most reliably achieved by a duplication technique, in which for the sake of maintaining stability, the occlusal and polished surfaces are preserved as in the original and only the fitting surfaces replaced to improve retention. Duplication techniques have developed rapidly of late and are now cheap and easy to use.[4] Alginate is the investment material of choice, being much cheaper than the alternative of silicone rubber and being equally accurate.[5] Originally the template of the denture to be duplicated was cast in either wax or acrylic resin. Both had problems. Wax has low strength, and adhesion of some impression materials to a wax base is poor. With acrylic resin, while its strength is valuable for chairside work, its toughness is disliked by technicians who have to remove the tooth part of the template, waxing on artificial teeth in its place. Fortunately, there is a compromise technique (see Appendix) which involves producing a template with a fitting surface of acrylic resin, the remainder being of wax. The composite structure satisfies the requirements of clinician and technician.

Another common clinical situation involving diminished adaptation with age arises when an elderly person with a few remaining teeth decides that enough have been lost to warrant replacement by a complete denture. In such cases the treatment of choice is always a transitional denture, when the period of habituation can be prolonged, and after adaptation to a partial denture the remaining teeth can be added one or two at a time. Partial dentures of simple design are first made to replace the missing teeth. They are designed to fit around the cervical margins of standing teeth to provide extra stability. After a period of adaptation, which can be as long as several months, the remaining teeth are added a few at a time. If the patient already possesses a partial denture which is well tolerated and of an appropriate design and material, the stages are simplified and addition of further teeth to it can take place at once.

Subsequently, transitional dentures require frequent review. Not only does addition of the remaining teeth take place over a prolonged time, with a period of re-adaptation following each extraction, but the patient's age usually contraindicates surgical reduction of bony undercuts. Frequent review is essential to preserve appearance, with progressive additions being made to the labial flange as resorption occurs.

The other personal details are less important, but with exceptions. Players of wind instruments are a special problem. Proper performance on their instrument depends on modifying the presssure and shape of a column of air in the mouth and oro-pharynx. Complete dentures make this difficult unless retention is ideal. Only limited help can be given to players of woodwind instruments, where the reed is held in the mouth. Necessarily, the dentures should be as retentive as possible, and in order to promote maximum muscular support of a prosthesis by the embouchure all facial surfaces of the denture should be concave. If the instrument demands a double lip embouchure (for example the oboe), displacing forces are applied anteriorly to both dentures, causing them to tilt posteriorly away from the denture-bearing surface (Fig. 1.1A and B). It has been reported that a removable spring added to the molar surfaces of a mandibular denture and positioned so as to give support to the maxillary denture, is helpful.[6] At times a special "embouchure denture" may be advised which provides mutual support to the mandibular and maxillary dentures in protrusion, by a system of interacting planes posteriorly.[7] The denture is used only for playing and is useless for other functions apart from aesthetics.

Players of the clarinet employ a single lip embouchure (Fig. 1.2). The mouthpiece is normally held in contact with the maxillary anterior teeth and for an edentulous player it is possible to modify it to give extra support to the maxillary denture. A piece of sticking plaster is

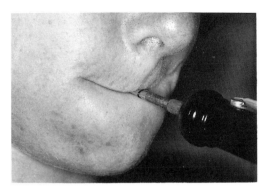

Fig. 1.1A Oboe being played. Note the powerful contraction of the circum-oral musculature.

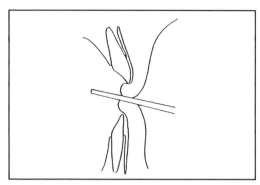

Fig. 1.1B Sagittal section of oboe embouchure.

added to the mouthpiece in such a position that it allows upwards and backwards pressure to be exerted on the incisal edges of the central incisors.

Unfortunately, brass instruments with their external mouthpiece provide the player with little opportunity to support dentures by means of the embouchure and although there are edentulous brass instrument players who can play well, few or none are of orchestral standard.

Actors and others in the public eye are reputed to make stringent demands as regards appearance, and a recent retirement or the death of a spouse can cause dramatic psychological changes and contraindicate all but temporary treatment. Finally, while the fact that a patient has travelled a considerable distance for treatment is likely to boost one's ego, it may be that they have exhausted the patience of all prosthodontists in their immediate vicinity and extra care should be taken over their assessment and treatment plan.

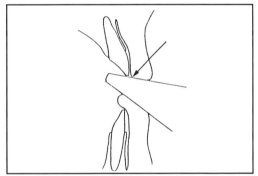

Fig. 1.2 Sagittal section of clarinet embouchure. If a complete maxillary denture is worn, support can be given by application of strip of adhesive plaster at the site marked with arrow to form a notch into which the maxillary central incisors fit.

The complaint

A problem that we have to be aware of at this stage is the nebulous complaint. We can be grateful that the majority of patients attend with a specific, identifiable fault, which in the case of

replacement dentures is usually pain, looseness, functional problems, or appearance. Patients of this type are rewarding to treat and correction of the defect ensures satisfaction. However, although the majority of patients have a specific complaint a small number do not, and are encouraged to attend by pressure from their family circle for treatment of problems of which they themselves are unaware. Treatment is then difficult because without an identifiable complaint there is no scale on which to judge improvement. A variation on this theme is when minor problems are magnified by self-concern or an isolated mode of life. Review of the personal details and perceptive questioning will reveal such complications. As a guide, remember that without a complaint there can be no cure, and if the patient is basically satisfied with his dentures it is difficult to make improvements.

Another patient to be assessed carefully is one who has worn his present dentures for some years and although they are still functional and problem-free, feels that taking into account the experiences of his friends, his dentures are now old enough to require replacement. Although such patients are usually stoical and will not complain if little or no improvement is made, they will be your wholehearted advocate in the future if after discussion minor improvements can be made at moderate expense by reline or addition.

Other patients have numerous vague complaints which disguise a disappointment with their appearance and an unvoiced hope that improvements in their looks and social acceptability will result from the provision of new dentures. Often their fundamental insecurity is confirmed by the medical history when they are found to be taking anxiolytic drugs. Such patients require time and care but with a full explanation are often prepared to accept the necessary treatment compromises.

One of the most difficult complaints to resolve by prosthodontic means is the burning mouth syndrome. Because medical treatment so frequently produces little in the way of improvement it is tempting to blame a prosthodontic fault, and because practitioners may well have slightly different ideas about the definition of the ideal complete denture it is relatively easy for the inexperienced prosthodontist to detect an "error". A complaint of burning mouth should be a sign to be extra vigilant. Some such cases do have a prosthodontic cause, namely lack of tongue space, lack of interocclusal space, or excessive levels of monomer in the resin. Suspicion should be aroused if the symptoms started soon after the provision of a new denture. On the other hand if the symptoms persist despite removing the denture from the mouth for several hours, replacement of the denture by another will be unlikely to produce a cure no matter how excellent the clinical and technical standards of work. Fortunately, recent investigations[8] into the classification and therapy of burning mouth syndrome hold hope for a more rational diagnosis and treatment for this troublesome complaint.

Three types of burning mouth were defined in the study; 1, where there are no symptoms on waking but burning begins and its severity increases during the day; 2, the burning persists throughout the day; and 3, there are symptom-free days and unusual sites (e.g. floor of the mouth or throat) are involved. In type 1 the aetiology was often found to be local in origin, but with types 2 and 3, anxiety and allergy, respectively, were encountered. Replacement of faulty dentures was helpful in about 25% of all cases, the main defects being lack of freeway space, restricted tongue space or overloading of tissues due to underextension of the base. These problems were found to be especially likely when the burning started following the recent provision of new dentures. Among non-denture causes, haematological deficiency, diabetes, candidal infection or xerostomia were commonly diagnosed.

Dental history

In a perfect world we would all keep our teeth for life, but if all the teeth have to be lost then ideally any patient attending for replacement of complete dentures should have been rendered edentulous at a comparatively early age, have adapted well to the change and have shown excellent tolerance by a history of uncomplicated denture replacement every 5 or so years. Compliant patients like this are quickly and easily satisfied but more infrequently come to us for attention because their numbers are diminishing. In their place are increasing numbers of denture cripples with a range of problems to overcome.

An underlying problem may be suspected if denture wearing is intermittent or dentures are frequently replaced. When an elderly patient has been rendered edentulous or the denture has been provided for the first time during retirement when lack of mental stimulus can make adaptation difficult, the dental history is often one of constant failure. The patient with a bag of dentures is a tribulation mentioned in all books on the subject and unfortunately still occasionally attends practitioners' surgeries. All too often the patient's problem is not of dental origin but is associated with a period of crisis in their life, or an unwillingness to face the realities of denture wear. Treatment is frustrating unless this is recognized, and referral for psychotherapy may be the only recourse. Referral for a specialist opinion may help to the extent that it vindicates the practitioner's original diagnosis and reassures the patient that everything possible is being done.

Not all patients with numerous sets of complete dentures are in the above category and careful assessment must be made, especially of those with a history of numerous replacement dentures provided over the last few years and associated with a prior period of satisfactory denture wear. Careful examination of the current denture should reveal a fault. When the patient has been rendered edentulous in the comparatively recent past, again causative factors can often be discovered – especially in younger patients – such as minimal interalveolar space or postural protrusion, which make denture provision difficult and can sometimes be linked with a history of denture fracture. In others spreading of the tongue may have reduced the space available for the denture. The chronology of tooth loss is then significant and the history might reveal that posterior teeth have been lost and remained unreplaced for many years, so allowing tongue spreading to occur. The position of optimum stability of artificial teeth then no longer coincides with the position once occupied by the natural teeth.

Even the degree of difficulty experienced during earlier extractions can be significant. When extractions have been difficult there is a greater chance that buccal bone has been fractured and lost, with irregularities and excess resorption of the alveolar process. Difficult extractions are also associated with retained root fragments and note must be made to ensure that a radiographic scan is prescribed.

Medical history

Few diseases are an absolute contraindication to provision of complete dentures. Broadly speaking, four types can cause problems, viz. those affecting the bone of the jaws and alveolar processes, those affecting the mucosa, those affecting muscle and denture control, and those affecting saliva production.

Diseases of the bone are unusual and are rarely encountered. In the case of Paget's disease of bone little can be done apart from replacing dentures if they have become ill-fitting. While it would be frustrating to repeatedly provide replacement dentures for a patient suffering from acromegaly and complaining of

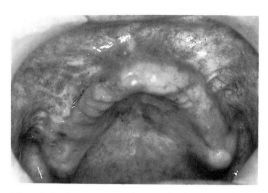

Fig. 1.3 Ten years after radiotherapy of the maxilla: enlarged superficial capillaries are still visible.

gradual loss of fit, it is unlikely that untreated cases of acromegaly will be encountered and if they are discovered they should be referred for treatment of the systemic condition before offering a prosthodontic service.

The complaint of sudden pain, swelling, and loss of fit of a denture is usually symptomatic of a local cause such as an infected residual cyst or retained root, but loss of fit over a period of a few months may be associated with an expanding neoplasm and should be treated with the greatest mistrust. Although hyperparathyroidism has been looked on with suspicion for many years, it is not responsible for rapid alveolar resorption.

Diseases of the mucosa are more common and aphthous ulcers, both minor and major, make denture wearers extremely uncomfortable because virtually all parts of the mouth come into contact with a denture during function. Other conditions such as atrophic lichen planus and pemphigoid are less common in the general population but relatively more common in the elderly. Some relief for all these conditions can be given by prescription of a topical steroid gel, and it goes without saying that great care must be taken to avoid errors in the occlusal

and jaw relationships. Discrepancies of this nature can cause any denture to exceed the limited tolerance of its supporting tissues.

Immediately following radiotherapy of the mouth the related mucosa becomes inflamed and tender and many post-radiotherapy cases remain permanently recognizable by the presence of permanently enlarged superficial capillaries (Fig. 1.3). Any necessary prosthodontic treatment can be done when the mucosal reaction has subsided, and a year is not an unreasonable time to wait. Needless to say, every attempt is made to ensure that the dentures are as atraumatic as possible and to minimize the risk of mucosal damage, or even osteo-radionecrosis, balanced articulation is advisable. When radiotherapy is associated with hyposalivation and pain due to lack of lubrication, artificial salivas are helpful.

More problems are likely to occur if a patient suffers from some types of neuromuscular complaint. Parkinson's disease, if advanced or poorly controlled, gives rise to tremor and facial rigidity, both causing difficulties when registering the jaw relationships. In addition, the patient's posture, which is often kyphotic with flexion of head and neck, makes access to the mouth difficult. The further complication of poor oral hygiene is only to be expected but it is often a surprise to find that despite some forms of medication (anticholinergic type, but not levodopa) having the side effect of causing hyposalivation, excess salivation and drooling are frequent. At times prescription of psychotherapeutic drugs to the elderly can have the side effect of tardive diskinesia, in which involuntary facial movements are so severe that no mandibular denture can be worn (Fig. 1.4).

Uncontrolled epilepsy can be a hazard for a denture wearer. There is not only the danger of breaking the denture during

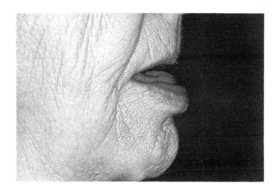

Fig. 1.4 Involuntary tongue protrusion in tardive dyskinesia causing the mandibular denture to be unstable.

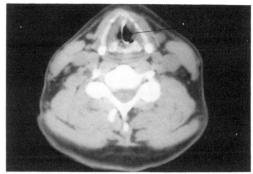

Fig. 1.5 CT scan of the larynx. The arrow indicates an impacted piece of denture hindering respiration.

a muscular spasm, but during a period of uncontrolled movement, dentures— especially fractured parts of dentures— can be inhaled. Although computerized tomographic scans will reveal pieces of acrylic resin (Fig. 1.5), normal radiographs will not.[9] An excellent case could be made for making radio-opaque all dentures for epileptics, whether well controlled or not, were a satisfactory denture resin of this type available.

Bell's palsy is usually a temporary disability, which is fortunate because it is difficult to improve the appearance by modifications to dentures. If the patient's maxillary denture is reasonably retentive a quick result is achieved by thickening the periphery of the denture in the canine region. The appearance at rest is improved but the deformity is immediately apparent on speaking and the lip often has a swollen appearance. A clear acrylic hook can be made which is attached to the canine and supports the affected lip at the corner, but it interferes with speech, is visible and causes maceration of the skin in contact with the hook. When the condition remains permanent a fascial graft is inserted or, in selected young patients, a nerve/muscle transplant from pectoralis minor.

Lack of saliva is a distressing condition and produces clinical problems which will be dealt with in later chapters. Few common diseases, apart from diabetes, have the potential to affect saliva flow directly, but it would be unusual for a patient's diabetes to be uncontrolled to the extent that dryness of the mouth was a complaint. Other diseases cause diminution of saliva flow and do so because their treatment involves the administration of drugs liable to cause hyposalivation as a side effect. A drug history is therefore essential. The drugs which often cause hyposalivation are numerous (Fig. 1.6) and of the associated conditions, anxiety states and depressive illness are commonest for which anxiolytics or antidepressants may be prescribed. In addition, many kinds can occasionally cause dry mouth either by themselves or in association with some other drug. The combination of methyl dopa and diuretic, as used to treat hypertension, is very potent.

A drug history is especially important because a history of psychotherapeutic drug treatment is one of the few useful indicators of possible difficulty in adapting to new dentures and, as mentioned above, treatment of the elderly with psychotherapeutic agents can cause tardive dys-

Type of drug	Examples
Anticholinergics	
(antispasmodic)	propantheline (*Pro-Banthine*)
(antiparkinsonian)	benzhexol (*Artane*)
Antihistamines and	chlorpheniramine (*Piriton*)
antinausea drugs	prochlorperazine (*Stemetil*)
Antidepressants	amitryptiline (*Tryptizol*)
	imipramine (*Tofranil*)
Systemic	salbutamol (*Ventolin*)
bronchodilators	terbutaline (*Brycanyl*)
Antipsychotics	chlorpromazine (*Largactil*)
	haloperidol (*Serenace*)
Antihypertensives	methyl dopa (*Aldomet*)
Diuretics	cyclopenthiazide (*Navidrex*)

In addition benzodiazopines, although infrequently causing dry mouth, are so commonly prescribed for depressive illness that their effect is significant.

Fig. 1.6 List of common drugs causing hyposalivation as a side effect. (Adapted from, Seymour, R.A. Dental pharmacology problems in the elderly. *Dental Update.* **15**:375–381, 1988.)

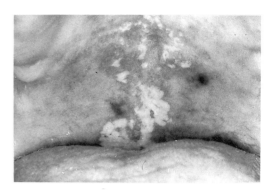

Fig. 1.7 Candidosis of the soft palate following frequent use of a salbutamol aerosol inhaler for relief of asthma.

kinesia which adversely affects a patient's ability to wear dentures.

Two further types of drug have complications of relevance to complete denture prosthodontics. Steroids and immuno-suppressives delay healing and make patients liable to local candidal infections, as do aerosol bronchodilators (selective beta2-adrenoreceptor stimulants) used for asthma relief (Fig. 1.7).

Examination

As with the assessment generally, it is tempting to rush this stage and proceed immediately to the examination of the mouth. Always act with restraint and first make a thorough extra-oral search.

Extra-oral examination

While all aspects of the extra-oral examination are important there are some of particular relevance to the prosthodontist. The extra-oral examination must include palpation of the regional lymph nodes and examination of the TMJs. Cancer of the mouth has a poor prognosis, and it would be negligent to miss any sign of it or, at a later stage, confuse it with an ulcer due to denture trauma. Pain and/or crepitus of the temporomandibular joints is very common. It would be remiss not to note their state of health or disease for fear the patient became aware of previously existing symptoms after prosthodontic treatment was complete, and assumed the new dentures to be the cause. It would reassure such a patient to know that temporomandibular symptoms had been noted and recorded before treatment had begun.

The salivary glands and any associated swellings are palpated. Painless swelling of the salivary glands can be associated with Sjögren's disease, an autoimmune condition in which enlargement of the salivary glands causes a reduction in saliva flow and dry mouth. An associated arthritis may make one suspect the condition but biopsy of the lip (to identify changes in the minor salivary glands) is needed for confirmation. Any facial asymmetry should be noted and the history reviewed to check if it is developmental or associated with trauma. Finally note any tremor, muscle weakness or abnormality of function or speech, again reviewing it in relation to the medical history.

At this stage the skeletal relationships of the jaws should be noted.The problems of the class III jaw relationship are well known. Where only a moderate skeletal discrepancy exists, good results can be expected when the anterior teeth are provided with an edge-to-edge relationship. The small degree of proclination of the maxillary anterior teeth needed to ensure incisal contact can usually be achieved in a well retained denture without destabilizing it. When the original skeletal discrepancy was marked and the original reverse overjet large, the difficulties of producing an aesthetic and functionally stable tooth arrangement will be so much the greater and a class III incisor relationship may have to be accepted as well as a posterior cross-bite. Thickenings of the maxillary labial periphery are often made to give additional lip support and make the horizontal discrepancy of the maxilla less obvious. If this course of action is taken, the operator must be prepared to make progressive reductions of the periphery at subsequent review stages if tissue tolerance is exceeded.

The gonial angle, or the angle between the posterior border of the ramus and the inferior border of the body of the mandible, is significant. It is associated with a class III jaw relationship, elongation of the lower third of the face, and sometimes a natural anterior open bite with incompetent lips. Recognition of a high gonial angle at this stage can save time later. It is often impossible to provide a

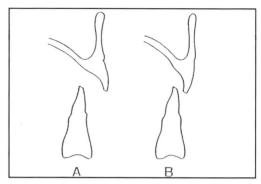

Fig. 1.8 Modification of the site of maxillary central incisors to provide lip support and improved appearance. A, incisors with excess overjet before modification. B, incisors retroclined to reduce overjet but maintain lip support.

functional incisor relationship unless the situation is recaptured which existed before the teeth were removed.

A class II jaw relationship has fewer insurmountable problems. The natural incisor relationship could have been either a div. i or div. ii. Either can be reproduced in a complete denture, but patients usually prefer the latter for its better appearance and reduced overjet. A considerable reduction of any excess overjet can be achieved, without compromising stability, by retroclining the maxillary incisor teeth so that the labial cervical margins remain in the normal position 8–10 mm in front of the palatine papilla and provide the lip support which would be absent if the incisor teeth were moved bodily lingually (Fig. 1.8). This is said to work best when the natural incisor relationship was class II div. ii, because hinge type masticatory movements are adopted during life and the habit of minimal forward translation means that interference of the anterior teeth does not occur.

Often in natural class II relationships the mandibular incisors are proclined to accommodate to the labial musculature. If retroclining the artificial maxillary incisors gives insufficient improvement in appearance to satisfy the patient, further reductions in the overjet can be tried by slightly proclining the mandibular incisors, the incisal tips then come into near normal relationship with the retroclined maxillary incisors and still fit in with the musculature of the lip and tongue. If bodily forward movement of the mandibular incisors is tried, it creates a pressure against the lower lip which leads to denture instability.

The problem with class II relationships which is most difficult to resolve, but only arises when immediate replacement of anterior teeth is contemplated, is the appearance of the mandibular incisors when the natural dentition shows a complete anterior overbite—often a result of overclosure following loss of posterior teeth. In order to preserve the original face height and still allow space for a maxillary denture base, the artificial mandibular incisors must be reduced in length. When the patient objects to the reduced amount of visible mandibular tooth and it is thought risky to alter the tooth positions, the only alternative is to make whatever decrease in freeway space is tolerable.

Note is made of any developmental or acquired abnormalities of lip posture. Establishment of aesthetic occlusal planes at the registration stage will depend on compromises between function and facial harmony. The anterior occlusal plane should generally parallel the interpupillary line which in turn is usually parallel to the line of the smiling upper lip. When the smiling upper lip is asymmetric and not parallel to the interpupillary line, an anterior occlusal plane parallel to the interpupillary line will be discordant unless the incisor line more or less follows the smiling lip line. On the same principle, to make any residual notching of a repaired cleft lip less noticeable a corresponding irregularity should be placed in the artificial teeth. A brief record in the notes now, on either of these points will ensure that memory does not fail at a later stage.

If evidence of angular cheilitis is seen it is normally indicative of an infection, either by *Candida albicans* or staphylococci. Swabs are taken of the fitting surface of the denture (to confirm the presence of *Candida albicans*), the commissures and the nares (in case the infection is being transmitted via the fingers). Once the responsible organism is identified an effective antibiotic can be prescribed. This will be combined with treatment of any identified denture stomatitis and must include instruction in oral and denture hygiene. Nystatin and amphotericin B are effective against *Candida albicans*, fusidic acid cream against staphylococci, and miconazole gel against both.

Angular cheilitis is frequently associated with lack of lip support and for permanent relief the natural lip contour has to be restored. When new dentures are provided care should be taken to site the maxillary central incisors correctly, so giving support for the upper lip and reducing the fold at the commissures. Thickening the denture base periphery in the maxillary incisor and canine regions does not draw the upper lip forwards and merely gives a swollen appearance to the lip.

The final stage is to make a preliminary check of the occlusal and rest face heights. Lack of interocclusal space is so often the cause of symptoms both simple and complex that this procedure must never be omitted.

Intra-oral examination

The intra-oral examination should proceed in an orderly fashion to ensure that no aspect is forgotten. A convenient routine is to begin with the soft tissues,

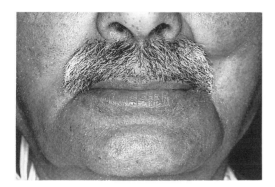

Fig. 1.9 Extra-oral appearance of submucous fibrosis. Tight fibrous bands have caused depressions of the left cheek.

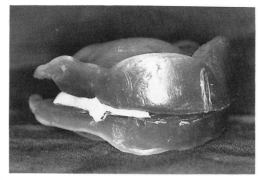

Fig. 1.10A Case of submucous fibrosis. The jaw relations have been recorded in permanent bases and located with silicone putty.

examining the cheeks, lips, tongue and floor of mouth in turn. Progress to the hard tissues, examining the palate, alveolar ridges and denture-bearing areas. Chart and examine any standing teeth, and finally examine any dentures.

Soft tissues

The range of systemic diseases with manifestations in the mouth is diverse enough to provide a career for specialists in oral medicine. From the point of view of complete denture prosthodontics there are relatively few conditions of the mucosa which complicate or contraindicate treatment. Apart from ulcerative conditions mentioned above in the history, which inhibit denture wear on account of the pain they cause, uncommon conditions such as submucous fibrosis and scleroderma cause problems by preventing access. In submucous fibrosis (Fig. 1.9), taut fibrous bands form in the cheeks, which limit the mouth opening and reduce the sulcus depth. When making complete dentures for the first time the initial difficulty is usually access for any necessary oral surgery. Later, primary impressions can be taken with drastically reduced stock trays. The available space

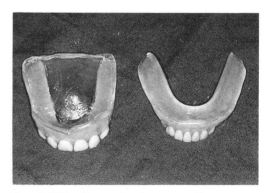

Fig. 1.10B Case of submucous fibrosis. The final dentures show limited extension due to reduction of the sulcus depth by fibrous bands.

constricts further with time and when replacement dentures are required the previous dentures are used as special trays and an impression made in fluid silicone, the patient positioning the "tray" himself. Acrylic resin permanent bases are made for the registration using a location technique which permits the two blocks to be removed separately and reassembled (Fig. 1.10A and B). A technique has also been described for making the maxillary denture in two interlocking halves,[10] but it would be difficult to make a mandibular denture in this way due to tongue interference.

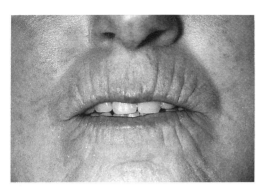

Fig. 1.11 Case of scleroderma. Complete dentures have recently been provided.

The prosthodontic problems of systemic sclerosis or scleroderma (an auto-immune condition) are similar and arise when the face is affected by the disease. The mouth has a drawn appearance, with a change taking place in the collagen of the lips rendering them stiff and inelastic (Fig. 1.11). Both submucous fibrosis and systemic sclerosis are progressive and ultimately make it impossible to place or remove any form of denture. Some help can be gained in the case of submucous fibrosis by dividing the fibrous bands, exercise, and the injection of steroids submucosally, although further deterioration is usual. The prognosis for scleroderma is similarly poor, although systemic steroids have an ameliorative effect.

A common local condition which causes difficulty not with access but with denture fracture, is enlarged fraenal attachments which in severe cases can unite the lips and cheeks with the crest of the ridge. When present the notch formed in the denture base causes stress concentration and the future denture will be liable to sudden fracture unless the fraenum is removed surgically prior to making dentures. In cases where surgery is impossible, due to age, phobia or medical condition, the patient can be warned that a metal base is needed.

While examining the soft tissues an assessment should be made of the amount of saliva. Saliva has diverse functions but the most important is to act as a lubricant and cleaner of the mouth and allow eating and speaking to be performed in comfort. When a complete denture is worn its retention depends on the presence of an intact saliva film. Where there is a deficiency of saliva, which may be caused by drug therapy, auto-immune disease or radiotherapy, not only are speech and eating more difficult and eased only by constant drinks of water, but denture retention is poor, oral hygiene difficult to maintain and mucosal infections common. In severe cases the mucosa will look and feel dry.

Saliva deficiency may be suspected if in the absence of other possible causes, the patient complains that he wakes at night at regular intervals to drink water. Lack of lubrication by saliva makes the mandibular denture-bearing area sore due to constant friction with the slightly mobile denture and the persistent pain may be misdiagnosed as a denture fault. When relief can be produced in no other way the mandibular denture is sometimes mistakenly relined with a silicone-rubber soft liner. The immediate effect is to increase the coefficient of friction between the denture and the mucosa and make the pain worse. Prescription of sialogogues has little place in the treatment of dry mouth for the alleviation of prosthodontic problems, and while sucking citrus sweets offers temporary help, more permanent relief is provided by prescription of an artificial saliva.[11] As an alternative, when the condition is mild, and soreness beneath the denture the only problem, a small amount of a liquid denture adhesive will act as a lubricant and can be applied to the fitting surface.

Before progressing to examine the

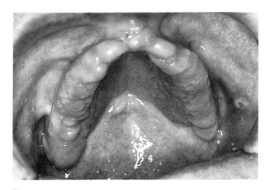

Fig. 1.12 Denture stomatitis associated with papillary hyperplasia of the palate.

Denture stomatitis

Denture stomatitis (or denture-associated candidosis or chronic atrophic candidosis), is caused by *Candida albicans* and occurs at some time in about two-thirds of the elderly denture-wearing population.[13] It can be classified into three distinct forms: I—discrete red areas beneath the maxillary denture; II—generalized redness of the entire maxillary denture-bearing area; and III—generalized redness associated with papillary hyperplasia (Fig. 1.12). Patients are not always aware of its presence and it belies its original name of denture sore mouth by rarely causing acute pain or soreness, although 28% of sufferers are aware of a burning or tingling sensation.[14] In the more severe forms patients may complain of a thickening or "succulent" feeling of the mucosa of the palate which is a consequence of papillary hyperplasia. The actual epithelial response is variable, although on average it is slightly thicker than normal[15] despite the alternative name for the condition of chronic atrophic candidosis. The underlying connective tissue, too, is thickened, and the enlarged blood vessels are visible through the mucosa and give rise to the red appearance.

In a recent review[16] it was claimed that while some type I cases are caused by denture trauma, types II and III are always associated with poor oral hygiene, which allows *Candida albicans* or a similar fungus to proliferate in the plaque formed on an unhygienic denture. That denture stomatitis rarely affects the mandibular denture may be due to the relatively poor retention and anatomical site of the latter. A constant slight flow of saliva over the fitting surface promoting cleanliness.

Endotoxins from the fungus cause the inflammation and permanently removing the dentures will eliminate the infection. This is not a form of treatment

alveolar processes and denture-bearing areas the tongue and floor of mouth are examined. If the patient has been without dentures for a considerable time, or if the mandibular posterior teeth were extracted some time ago without a partial denture being provided and the patient has become accustomed to using only the natural anterior teeth for eating, spreading of the tongue might have occurred into the space once occupied by the teeth. A mandibular denture with the teeth in the normal bucco/lingual position will be unstable or the tongue constriction may result in soreness or burning sensations. Some form of neutral zone recording can help ensure a pain-free, stable prosthesis[12] (see Chapter 2). If a previous complete mandibular denture is unstable because it constricts the tongue, indentations in the lateral border of the tongue corresponding to the site of the artificial posterior teeth are diagnostic.

Alveolar processes and denture-bearing areas

The palate, alveolar ridges and denture-bearing area are inspected and palpated in turn. Certain conditions of special interest to the prosthodontist may be encountered.

which is socially acceptable to most patients and we are therefore obliged to treat the candidal infection by alternative means. *Candida albicans* is not a strongly pathogenic organism and the presence of denture stomatitis may be indicative of a debilitating systemic disease, e.g. anaemia, diabetes or immunocompromising condition. The appropriate tests should be made when particularly florid or resistant forms are encountered.

For the dentist the local clinical consequences of the disease are few. Some small degree of stability will be lost by placing a denture on an inflamed surface, and retention may be affected if the degree of mucosal inflammation changes between the time of taking the impressions and delivery of the denture. When the disease is discovered the reasons for treating it are principally medical. The elderly are susceptible to candidal infections, especially if a degree of immunological incompetence exists or if, as a result of drug therapy, the immune response is diminished. They may then develop candidosis of the lungs, gastrointestinal tract or bloodstream by dissemination from an oral source. Denture stomatitis should be treated effectively before dentures are replaced, and suitable instructions given to ensure that it does not recur.

The first step is adequate diagnosis, which can be difficult for the practitioner when microbiological help is unavailable. Although the appearance of types II and III is almost pathognomonic, swabs of the fitting surface of the maxillary denture, tongue and the denture-bearing area must be taken (imprint samples and impression cultures require even more specialised arrangements).[17] Organisms are most reliably isolated from the fitting surface of the denture. After culture the disease is confirmed not by the identification of individual organisms but by culture of large numbers of colony-forming units.

Type I cases may simply be due to mucosal damage by the denture. If candida is not isolated, then after relief of the trauma (usually by application of a temporary soft lining) new dentures can be made. In all cases, when candida is isolated treatment begins with a demonstration and explanation of the cause of the disease to the patient. Improved oral hygiene must be encouraged and in mild cases is the only treatment required. Effective fungicidal agents are hypochlorite solution and chlorhexidine, and the patient can be advised to soak the denture in either of these solutions overnight. Complications are few and are principally the unpleasant taste of a denture which has been soaked for a prolonged period in hypochlorite, and the staining which accompanies immersion of acrylic in chlorhexidine. If after 6 weeks the inflammation has resolved, oral hygiene has improved and swabs show lack of fungi, new dentures can be made.

This regime also works with types II and III if patients will comply with instructions. When they refuse to remove the denture at night or when in severe cases it is suspected that the tongue is acting as a reservoir, treatment with antifungal agents is best. Nystatin is effective but has an unpleasant taste. Even in the form of flavoured pastilles the taste is too strong for some patients. Miconazole oral gel is the treatment of choice, with 2–3 cm of the ointment being extruded onto the fitting surface of the denture four times per day. A little can also be applied to an associated angular cheilitis. The ointment is pleasant tasting (unlike other topical antifungal agents) and has the additional effect of acting as a denture adhesive and improving the fit of the denture. Recent work has even shown that in cases where patients have not complied with conventional therapy, miconazole base can provide effective treatment when implanted into the denture in the form of a sustained release device.[18]

To ensure success, any form of treatment must be prolonged beyond the time at which clinical resolution of the condition has occurred. Most of the causative fungi can exist in a spore phase in which they resist treatment, and an extra few weeks must be allowed to permit spores to germinate and be killed. Six weeks is considered an adequate treatment time. For those with facilities available a more accurate assessment of the progress of treatment can be made by cleaning the denture in sterile water in an ultrasonic bath, culturing and counting the number of organisms removed in the sonicate.[19] By repeating the procedure at subsequent reviews the rate of resolution of the disease can be monitored and the point determined at which the organism is eliminated from the mouth.

Despite careful treatment, some patients who show an immediate improvement which is maintained for some months, later suffer recurrence, whether due to lack of oral hygiene or some systemic factor. If tests show no undiagnosed systemic condition, a modern systemic antifungal agent such as fluconazole can be prescribed. The alternative, ketoconazole, should not be prescribed without careful consideration and bearing in mind that liver damage has been reported as a side effect.

Following elimination of the infection and its associated inflammation any papillary hyperplasia will become less marked. If the patient remains concerned about the hyperplasia, residual enlargement can be removed surgically.

Palatal tori
Examination of the hard palate may reveal the presence of a palatal torus. The covering of thin mucoperiosteum over such a structure does not give the resilient support found over the alveolar processes. As a consequence, under masticatory loads there is a local increase in pressure and pain, with flexing of the denture. Treatment involves relief of the denture over the torus. While a spacer of foil can be incorporated before processing, the spacing that results is entirely arbitrary and further reduction at the insertion stage will probably be required. Very large tori of this type can be treated by surgical removal but surgery is best reserved for when all else fails. Few patients relish the prospect of surgery; the experience of having a large torus removed is most unpleasant unless carried out as an in-patient under general anaesthesia. Perforation of the palate is not an uncommon surgical complication and prolonged post-operative pain can make denture wearing difficult.

Undercuts
When examining the edentulous ridges make note of any areas of undercut and whether the undercut exists only in relationship to a vertical path of withdrawal or whether it can, like many undercuts found in the anterior maxilla, be eliminated by altering the path of withdrawal. When a decision is difficult study models may be needed to provide a reliable answer. An identified undercut may be either of soft tissue or partly of hard tissue. When partly of hard tissue (and frequently when entirely soft tissue), the denture will not enter the undercut without causing pain and ideally the undercut should be eliminated surgically before starting to make impressions. Alternatively, to avoid the inevitably less precise chairside reduction of the alveolar surface of the denture flange at the delivery stage and to prevent treatment being fur-

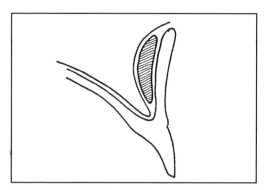

Fig. 1.13 Diagram illustrating the site for support of the labial flange of a denture by a hydroxyapatite implant. Shaded area—implant.

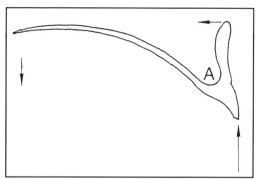

Fig. 1.14 Diagram of the forces applied to a maxillary denture during mastication. Arrows indicate directions of displacement. A, axis of rotation.

ther prolonged, undercuts on the working model can be blocked out prior to processing. It is sometimes assumed that in the case of bilateral undercuts in the tuberosity region only one undercut need be reduced, the other acting as an aid to retention, and the effect is often illustrated by a diagrammatic coronal section through the tuberosity region. Unless the maxillary alveolar process is substantially of soft tissue, this is an over-simplification. In three dimensions the shape of the alveolus will provide anterior guide planes which prevent rotational paths of insertion and removal.

Sometimes it is possible to eliminate undercuts not by removing bone but by augmenting the undercut area with hydroxyapatite particles inserted via a surgical tunnel. The indications are few but it can be a useful and relatively atraumatic operation when a deep maxillary labial undercut exists. By filling the space labial to the undercut, support is given to the labial flange of the denture, allowing it to resist rotation in a sagittal plane and provide more retention (Fig. 1.13). Following the operation, migration of implanted particles is prevented by the patient wearing their original denture but having the labial flange adjusted to fit against the implanted site.

Although dentures will enter small soft-tissue undercuts it should not be assumed that undercuts of this type can be recorded with an inelastic impression material. Their presence causes technical difficulties because the model cast from the impression is a "hard tissue" undercut. Models are frequently damaged during withdrawal of an inelastic material, especially if zinc oxide impression material is used and the period of warming prior to removal of the impression from the cast is too short to allow adequate softening. It follows that if undercuts are identified, then to ensure accurate work, an elastic material is always the material of choice.

Atrophic fibrous anterior maxilla

Atrophic fibrous ridges are common in the anterior maxillary region, especially in patients with retained mandibular anterior teeth, although the condition appears to occur whether or not a partial denture is worn.[20] It is easy to hypothesize a cause. The direction of the applied force of mastication causes slight rotation of the denture around the anterior maxillary alveolus and pressure of the distally rotating anterior flange against the labial plate of bone causes resorption (Fig.

1.14). The shearing forces applied to the mucoperiosteum by friction with the base during rotation then result in fibrous hyperplasia. In time much of the anterior maxilla may be replaced by fibrous tissue with poor denture-supporting properties. Whenever the patient incises, the pad of fibrous tissue is compressed and upward movement of the maxillary denture anteriorly causes downward displacement posteriorly, with loss of retention in the post dam region.

Treatment may be of two types, the conservative and the surgical. Conservative treatment involves judicious selection of impression materials and technique, and will be dealt with in Chapter 2. The techniques outlined are designed to ensure maximal retention during non load-bearing function—such as speaking —and rely on the hope that when retention is lost during mastication, the balancing contact of the opposed occlusal surfaces provides extra stability. While popular, the techniques are relatively unsuccessful in advanced cases.

The surgical options are more varied. The simplest is to excise the soft tissue, an operation which leaves an adequately firm residual base for denture support but one which is reduced in size and lacks all antero-posterior resistance to movement. The maxillary denture will now tend to be displaced anteriorly during mastication. A more useful alternative is to augment the alveolar ridge with a biocompatible bone substitute such as hydroxyapatite. Hydroxyapatite originally came in three forms, rounded dense particles, dense blocks, or porous blocks. Particles are inserted with a syringe through a vertical midline incision. To allow adequate space for the particles, subperiosteal and submucosal tunnels are dissected and joined.[21] A pre-formed splint or temporary denture is needed to prevent particle migration. Blocks can be inserted at open operation in the same way,[22] but unless there is sufficient thickness of soft tissue over them they tend to ulcerate through and become infected. Porous blocks are preferred by many surgeons because they are easier to cut to shape pre-operatively, but a recent communication[23] has drawn attention to their tendency to exfoliate following suspected infection of their internal spaces.

Surgical options appear to be the treatment of choice but they have disadvantages. Whichever method is used, perforation of the tunnel or flap is common despite the apparent thickness of the mucoperiosteum, due to the deeply cleft nature of the fibrous tissues. To prevent migration of the particles a temporary denture has to be first made on a model which has been modified to represent the ridge after augmentation. The temporary denture is worn for approximately 6 weeks or until the ridge is adequately firm to allow support of a permanent denture. During this period, instructions must be given for the patient to avoid hard foods and preferably wear the temporary denture for appearance only.

A more recently developed form of hyrdoxyapatite is one which is carveable and comprises dense particles surrounded by a collagen matrix.[24] Straight or curved, carveable rods are implanted beneath a lingually based mucoperiosteal flap at open operation. The operation is usually associated with sulcus deepening and the flap extended into the lip, where a section of the mucosa is mobilized and sutured to the periosteum of the buccal sulcus. If the operation is performed under general anaesthesia, a temporary denture made on an augmented model can be retained by a stainless steel palatal screw. A week later the screw is removed, and 6 weeks after that a replacement denture made.

All operations of this type involving the implantation of particulate hydroxyapatite, with or without a collagen matrix, suffer a considerable degree of loss of gained ridge height post-operatively. As much as 20% is lost over the first year.

Enlarged ridges
The usual consequence of enlarged alveolar ridges is lack of interalveolar space. The commonest type encountered is fibrous enlargement of the maxillary tuberosity, and it is impossible to design satisfactory dentures when, with the mandible in the rest position, contact or near contact occurs between the enlarged tuberosity and the retromolar pad. Surgical reduction of the superfluous fibrous tissue is indicated. After removal of a wedge of tissue over the crest of the tuberosity, the edges are undermined and sutured across the defect. If a complete denture is being worn, the space produced is occluded with a tissue conditioner/soft liner to preserve the fit during the period prior to denture replacement.

When the ridges are generally enlarged the expansion is usually bony rather than fibrous and the problems more acute. The operation for ridge reduction is much more prolonged and involves removal of bone from the entire surface of the alveolus. If, to avoid a prolonged operation, it is intended to reduce either the mandible or maxilla only, then from the point of view of aesthetics the maxilla should be chosen. An over-large maxillary alveolus gives insuperable problems with appearance. Either the teeth have to be reduced in length to an unacceptable degree, or the occlusal plane has to be so low that the patient will object to the amount of tooth showing.

Few elderly patients are prepared to undergo a ridge reduction operation, and so long as actual contact between the ridges does not occur a more conservative approach is undertaken to avoid the problems of denture fracture which in-

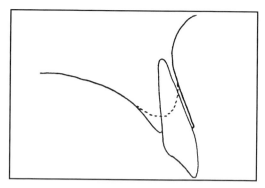

Fig. 1.15 Diagrammatic representation of the resorption pattern in the maxillary central incisor region. The dotted line indicates surface of alveolus after extraction and resorption.

variably follow the insertion of an inadequately thick prosthesis. Cast cobalt/chromium bases are prescribed, especially for the mandibular denture which is particularly liable to fracture. Enlarged mandibular ridges are often undercut and because a metal base will not enter a bony undercut, it can be designed to cover only the lingual surface of the alveolus anteriorly, passing forwards only as far as the ridge crest. This has the advantage that maximum space is left on the labial surface of the bone so that relatively normal sized mandibular incisors can be used.

Atrophic ridges
The stability of a complete denture depends to a considerable extent on a substantial residual, bony, alveolar ridge. The pattern of resorption which takes place when the teeth have been extracted is characteristic for each jaw. In the maxilla resorption takes place principally from the labial and buccal aspects. This is to be expected because the labial and buccal cortical plates are thinner than the lingual cortical plates and when resorption occurs the thinner plate will be resorbed more readily (Fig. 1.15).

Hence the resorbed edentulous maxillary alveolus is smaller antero-posteriorly and bucco-lingually than when the teeth were present, with a general movement of the residual ridge lingually.

In the mandible the pattern of alveolar bone loss is more complex and while in the incisor region the labial plate is slightly thinner than the lingual plate, in the premolar region the thicknesses are approximately equal and in the molar region the buccal plate becomes much thicker where it is buttressed by the external oblique ridge which increases in bulk towards the third molar region. Consequently, while in the incisor region the residual ridge shows a small lingual movement, in the premolar region the residual ridge occupies the same position as when the natural teeth were present, and in the molar region the residual ridge lies further bucally than the dentate ridge. The jaws also differ in the gross amount of bone lost. It has been shown that vertical alveolar bone loss in the mandible exceeds that in the maxilla by a factor of four.[25] The reason is not yet clear, nor can it be explained why in rare cases severe alveolar bone loss may affect only the maxilla.

For many patients the standard pattern of resorption is modified by the trauma accompanying tooth loss. When substantial amounts of buccal bone are removed either inadvertently or in the course of surgical removal of teeth, local bone loss is greater than expected. Denture wearing in itself does not appear to have a significant effect on resorption. Because it has been difficult to identify sufficiently large groups of non-denture wearers, investigations into this aspect have usually compared a group of subjects wearing their dentures at night with another group who do not.[26] With this qualification, to date no prospective clinical trial has been able to relate denture wearing with the extremes of alveolar bone loss. Although many practitioners will have encountered individual cases where a prominent residual maxillary alveolus is associated with a denture lacking a labial flange, and others in which extreme loss of bone in the mandibular premolar region accompanies prolonged denture wearing, it is difficult to prove that the two factors are causally related. In the former case the lack of labial flange may have been originally associated with an even larger and more prominent alveolus and in the latter the patient may have been one of those predisposed to extreme bone loss.

Rate of bone loss has been studied exhaustively. While the amount of loss varies from person to person, with some people suffering very little, the rate of loss is greatest immediately after extraction, becoming gradually less with time. Although it is customary to replace immediate dentures approximately 1 year after insertion when it is assumed that the majority of bone loss is over and the ridges are relatively stable, bone loss continues throughout life at a gradually decreasing rate until finally all alveolar bone is lost. It would therefore be more rational to wait longer than a year before making permanent dentures if resorption is seen to be rapid. For the same reason, although it is customary to recommend replacement of complete dentures at 5-year intervals, some patients are aware of a deterioration of fit after a year or so,[27] and while patients with slow resorption will need dentures to be replaced only after several years, a yearly review would be more appropriate for the majority. For the sake of maintaining the residual alveolar ridge a case may be made for retaining healthy teeth as long as possible.

A problem caused by extreme alveolar loss has been mentioned earlier when reference was made to the case of the

fibrous anterior maxilla, when denture
instability was the main problem. This
condition apart, the more intractable
problems of alveolar atrophy tend to concern the mandible. Generally the atrophic
mandible does not appear to be as predisposed to fibrous change as the maxilla
and denture problems are related more to
pain and looseness. Loss of mandibular
bone causes lack of denture resistance to
antero-posterior and lateral displacing
forces, a condition which may well be
compounded by any earlier difficulties
encountered in the clinic when trying to
locate special trays and registration blocks
accurately against flat atrophic man-
dibles. As a general rule, to avoid displacement caused by cuspal interference
and to preserve occlusal stability, flat
cusped teeth should be prescribed when
alveolar atrophy has occurred although
occlusal schemes for non-anatomic teeth
have their own problems (see Chapter 4).

Loss of alveolar bone in the premolar
region may be enough to cause the mental foramen to be situated on the crest of
the ridge in which exposed position it is
traumatized by the denture and becomes
a source of pain. When radiographs confirm the superficial position of the mental foramen the simplest remedy is to
relieve the denture over the palpable
neurovascular bundle. Relief by foiling
the model is rarely accurate or sufficient
and only adjustment of the base at the
chairside can guarantee effective pain
relief. All too often the pain is misdiagnosed and assumed to be due to buccal
overextension. Reduction of the base
then causes the denture to be less retentive. Rarely, intractable pain from this
cause may be rectified by surgical displacement of the neurovascular bundle
towards the lower border of the mandible. The post-operative complication of
permanent anaesthesia is common and
the patient must be adequately counselled

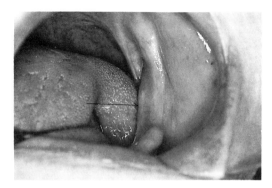

Fig. 1.16 Atrophic mandible with an arrow indicating the prominent mylohyoid ridge.

before embarking on such a course.

On the lingual surface of the body of
the mandible lies the mylohyoid line or
ridge which provides the mandibular
insertion of the mylohyoid muscle. The
mylohyoid line runs from the digastric
fovea at the midline, passes upwards and
backwards to the third molar region and
ends about 7 mm below the lingual crest
of the dentate ridge. In the second and
third molar region lingual resorption can
cause the mylohyoid ridge to become
prominent and form the medial boundary of the alveolar process (Fig. 1.16).
Extensions of the denture base over this
region may be painful. Recognition of
the cause of pain, associated with removal
of the denture base over the prominent
edge, will bring relief, but inevitably the
stabilizing influence of any extension of
the base medial to the mylohyoid ridge
might be lost. When there is pain from
this source and maximum medial extension is desired the attachment of the
mylohyoid muscle to the distal 1 cm or so
of the mylohyoid line can be excised and
the prominence of the ridge itself
reduced.

Treatment of the atrophic mandibular
ridge to improve denture stability means
increasing ridge height either relatively
or absolutely. A relative increase in ridge

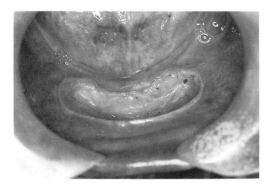

Fig. 1.17 Sulcus deepening procedure confined to the mandibular anterior region.

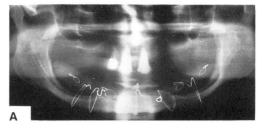

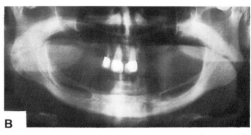

Fig. 1.18 Panoramic radiograph of atrophic mandible. A, immediately after augmentation with rib. B, 3 years later, following further resorption.

height is made by surgical deepening of the sulcus, an operation which depends for its success on covering the exposed surface with mucosa or skin and maintaining the acquired depth of sulcus against scar contraction by a splint or extension to the denture. During the healing phase the appliance is retained in place by circum-alveolar wires. Later a new, permanent denture is made. Sulcus deepening operations are more common in the mandible and to avoid damage to the mental nerve can be partial in extent and involve only the labial sulcus (Fig. 1.17). Paradoxically, the operation tends to work best in the case of maxillary sulcus deepening where, due to the pattern of alveolar resorption, it is less often needed.

Alternatively, an absolute increase in ridge height can be made. A number of materials have been used in the past including autogenous bone, a variety of polymers, and hydroxyapatite. Use of autogenous bone has the disadvantage that it is subject to resorption and any increase in ridge height is ultimately lost (Fig. 1.18). Synthetic polymers are stable but not being truly biocompatible and being incapable of uniting with bone, have tended to exfoliate. Hydroxyapatite is the most popular material to date and

for mandibular augmentation is usually used in the form of particles.[28] Although successful, the operation has complications. The gained ridge height is always less than expected and a sulcus deepening procedure is often needed later. Also, particulate forms tend to migrate with loss of gained ridge height—as witnessed by the numerous "spill prevention" remedies in the literature—and considerable particle loss can occur through the incision lines. Mental anaesthesia is a recognized complication following damage to the inferior dental nerve as it emerges from the mental foramen.

For this reason a new operation for localized augmentation has been recently developed which is applicable to those cases in which only a small degree of ridge augmentation is needed, and that in the premolar region.[29] The ideal patient is one with a history of successful mandibular denture wear in the past, but one for whom stability has decreased of late, following resorption of the remnants of the alveolar process. Minimal trauma is involved. The two-stage operation can be performed under local anaesthesia, and is suitable for the type of elderly patient the prosthodontist tends to deal with. Equally importantly, it can be performed by the general practitioner who, while needing a moderate amount of surgical training, possesses the prosthodontic skills needed to ensure best results.

Before any surgery is performed, impressions are made of the edentulous ridge, models cast and the premolar region built up to the required height in wax. The wax addition is removed and cast twice in surgical grade silicone before one cast is replaced in position on the model and the other sterilised. At a preliminary operation, and following use of chlorhexidine mouthrinses for a week, submucosal tunnels are raised on the lingual side of the alveolus from vertical incisions in the canine region and taken back to the retromolar pads. Subperiosteal tunnels are developed beneath the original tunnels, taken lingually and buccally and the roof incised over the ridge crest to unite them both. Into the spaces created the sterilized silicone spacers are inserted and the incision closed (Fig. 1.19).

While the preliminary operation is taking place the patient's mandibular denture is adjusted to fit loosely over the original model plus the spare silicone spacers, and when the operation is complete, the modified denture tried into the mouth and an accurate fit ensured by lining with a relatively elastic temporary soft liner such as Coe-Soft (Coe Labs Inc., Chicago, USA). A week or so later the soft liner is replaced by a tougher temporary liner such as Total-Soft (Stratford-Cookson Co., W. Hempstead, USA). Three weeks after the original operation, when a fibrous capsule has formed around the silicone spacers, the patient is recalled

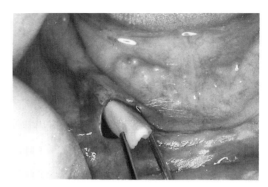

Fig. 1.19 Silicone spacer being placed into a subperiosteal tunnel.

and the spacers removed after remaking the original access incisions. Particulate hydroxyapatite is injected into the fibrous tissue lined tunnel and following closure of the incision the denture can be inserted. The developed shape of the fitting surface prevents migration of the hydroxyapatite particles. Six weeks later the modified dentures are replaced. Some loss of ridge height occurs over the following 6 months and the patient is recalled for reline of the denture after this time.

A more drastic, and at the same time more effective, method of increasing denture retention is by means of an implant. A variety of types of implant have been developed over the last few decades, most of which have suffered from a high rate of failure. The subperiosteal frames popular in the 60s and 70s suffered from infection which tracked down from the intra-oral part to the epithelium-encapsulated frame. Subsequent removal of the frame was prolonged and difficult. Successful dental implants followed from the work of Brånemark who developed the critical techniques which depend for their success on careful diagnosis and minimal damage to bone (Fig. 1.20). The well documented technique involves osseointegration of buried titanium fix-

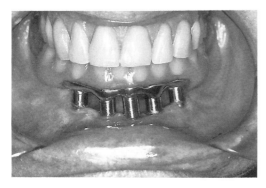

Fig. 1.20 Complete mandibular denture supported on osseointegrated titanium structures.

tures, with superstructures being placed on the fixtures only when integration is complete.[30] More recently, a large number of Brånemark-type, titanium implant systems have been developed which are based on the original work. While popular, none of these newer systems can provide the long-term research background of the originals. Many patients receiving implants can be expected to live for 30 or more years. It is therefore only sensible to ensure that the implant system of choice has a comparably long history of recorded, successful use.

Denture-associated trauma
Examination of the denture-bearing tissues of a patient who has worn complete dentures for some time may reveal a number of pathological changes which must be treated before new dentures can be made. With the passage of time alveolar resorption continues inexorably and an originally well fitting denture gradually loses its accurate fit. This is most obvious in the mandible because mandibular alveolar resorption is more pronounced. In time, with removal of the residual ridge the denture remains supported only by contact of the flanges with the basal bone. The increased stress applied to the intervening soft tissues can

cause a variety of responses. If the stress is enough to damage the integrity of the mucosal coverage, an ulcer results. Pain follows infection of the exposed surface and the patient usually attends to seek help. Less severe stress, insufficient to destroy the integrity of the mucosa, causes a hyperplastic reaction. Either hyperkeratosis of the denture-bearing area occurs, or else hyperplasia of the underlying connective tissue with production of a denture granuloma.

Before starting to make new dentures it is necessary to treat all signs of denture trauma, and remove all pathological swellings whether inflammatory or hyperplastic. Ulceration and keratinization are easily treated by removing the traumatizing section of denture base. However in most old, ill-fitting dentures the action is temporary and further damage occurs again at a different site. To ensure that the denture-bearing area remains healthy until new dentures are ready, and certainly until new working impressions have been made, a temporary soft liner is useful.

Modern temporary soft liners form part of a larger group of dental materials which includes the tissue conditioners and the functional impression materials. They are usually provided in the form of a powder and liquid. The powder is poly (butyl methacrylate), and the liquid a mixture of plasticizers, usually dibutyl phthalate and ethanol. One popular soft liner (Coe-Soft) also contains benzyl salicylate, an aromatic oil present in some sun-tan lotions and detergents, which is added to improve the mixing and handling properties.[31] When set, the temporary soft liners form visco-elastic gels which range in their properties from the more fluid (e.g. Visco gel, De Trey Dentsply Ltd., Weybridge, England) to the more elastic (e.g. Coe-Soft). The differences in properties are primarily due to differences in the initial powder/liquid ratio and, to some extent, judicious modification of the powder/liquid ratio of one's favourite brand can provide it with a range of properties wide enough to reproduce most of the various proprietary makes, even including the less elastic and more fluid functional impression materials.

After mixing an appropriate amount of temporary soft liner it is applied to the fitting surface of the denture, placed in the patient's mouth and allowed to gel under slight occlusal pressure from the opposing denture. All temporary soft liners are very adhesive to denture base resins and to prevent the material sticking to unwanted sites, a lubricant (silicone or coco oil) is provided. Once the material has set—a process which is purely physical gelation, no chemical polymerization is involved—the denture can be removed and surplus liner trimmed from the periphery with a scalpel. If on inspection the denture is seen to perforate the soft liner, a further layer is applied in the same way as before until the coating over the fitting surface is seen to be intact. It must be remembered that temporary soft liners have a clinical life which varies according to the conditions in the mouth but is, at most, measured in weeks. They cannot be used for long-term therapy and after they have been applied an appointment must always be made for review and more permanent treatment. With the very adhesive types it is also an advantage to reserve their use to appliances which will not have to be further modified or adapted. If they are used as a temporary measure before a permanent reline, the time occupied in removing the liner prior to making the reline impression may make the process uneconomical. Care must be taken over the cleaning of soft liners. Damage is easily done by mechanical methods and when certain immersion cleansers are used the physical properties of some soft liners deteriorate rapidly.[32]

The clinical life of a temporary soft liner is determined by the rate at which the plasticizers leach out. Where a more prolonged (but still not permanent) action is required, another material has been developed, the chairside-curing reline materials (e.g. Total). These are provided in a hard and soft form, the physical properties of the hard resembling denture base and those of the soft resembling a stiff soft liner. The materials set by a room-temperature, autopolymerizing process, the liquid containing mono (butyl methacrylate) and the powder, poly (butyl methacrylate). To ensure adhesion, the surface they are to be attached to must be primed with an acrylic monomer. The softness of the soft form is enhanced by incorporation of a plasticizer, which by reason of its high molecular weight diffuses out only very slowly. Both are exothermic on setting and for that reason, once the initial gel has taken place, final cure must take place outside the mouth. The chairside-reline materials are particularly useful for relining immediate dentures, when their longer clinical life allows review appointments to be spaced by months rather than weeks. The materials are not permanent and while fulfilling a most useful role, will ultimately deteriorate by discolouration and loss of their adhesive bond.

The denture-bearing tissues respond initially to moderate stress by keratinization and small white areas of keratinization are common beneath dentures more than a few months old. Chronic mechanical trauma excites a hyperplastic response from the underlying connective tissue and a denture granuloma, or area of denture-induced hyperplasia forms. Such soft tissue enlargements are usually seen at the periphery of the denture, either where the pressure is greatest following alveolar resorption or where an overexten-sion of the denture base has been present *ab initio* but because the patient's pain threshold is high or the damage not great enough to cause pain, they have not returned for adjustment. Classically, the tissue enlargement has a bifid form with the denture periphery separating the two lobes. When small, the internal lobe remains beneath the periphery of the den-ture until at last it grows large enough to slip to the outside and join the outer lobe, where it remains and a new internal granuloma forms beneath the original point of trauma. Ultimately the newly developing granuloma will become large enough to be displaced outwards in its turn. In time several granulomata form in succession, the resulting swelling hav-ing a lobulated appearance, each divi-sion representing the groove originally occupied by the denture periphery.

Treatment of denture granulomata is begun by relieving the denture at the point where the tissues are being trauma-tized, and if necessary applying a tempo-rary soft liner. A considerable degree of resolution of the swelling takes place as inflammation subsides both at the point of trauma and within the folds of the hyperplastic mass. Some clinicians have reported that merely removing the cause of trauma can produce resolution of small denture granulomata (although this has not been the writer's experience). If a substantial denture granuloma still remains after initial treatment, surgical removal is indicated.

Methods of removal of denture granu-lomata differ according to the nature of the underlying tissue.[33] If only attached mucosa is affected, removal will result in little subsequent shrinkage of the denture-bearing area and the denture granuloma can be removed by simple excision, cryosurgery or carbon dioxide laser. If the granuloma extends into the sulcus and involves alveolar mucosa there is a danger that loss of sulcus depth will fol-low the operation because any scar tissue formed will contract as it matures. When surgical excision of a lesion of this type is carried out the exposed connective tis-sues must be covered after undermining and mobilizing the adjacent mucosa. With a large lesion a split-skin graft can be placed over the raw area but involves an additional operation. For this reason laser surgery, which appears to result in the formation of less scar tissue and cor-respondingly less shrinkage, is becoming more popular. Laser treatment has the additional advantage that post-operative pain is less pronounced.

The V-shaped maxilla
Apart from the changes which follow resorption, the maxillary denture-bearing area may be of a shape which is not con-ducive to good support. While the square-shaped maxillary alveolus is well shaped for denture support, the V-shaped alveo-lus is notorious for the poor retention that often follows. The cause of this is not difficult to find. Following polymeriz-ation of the denture resin, shrinkage occurs towards those areas where the exotherm is greatest and which cure first, *viz.* the thicker parts incorporating the denture teeth.[34] Polymerization contrac-tion is compensated for by slight shrink-age of the entire palate, which by reason of its curvature produces a small gap between the denture base and the palate (for which the post dam is intended to compensate). When the palate is V-shaped, shrinkage is concentrated at the apex of the V instead of being distributed widely over a gentle curve. The poor fit is made worse in function because stress is also concentrated at this site[35] and during mastication the flexing of the palate and imperfect contact with the underlying tis-

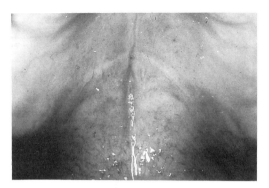

Fig. 1.21 Central longitudinal fissure of the palate causing the symptom of lack of retention.

sues causes loss of peripheral seal over the post dam region.

A problem also exists if there is a central longitudinal fissure of the soft tissues of the palate extending across the junction of hard and soft palate (Fig. 1.21), but then the lack of retention is because the knife-edge extension of the denture base into the fissure is removed by the technician who suspects a possible source of trauma. The solution is to complete the denture then add a functional post dam in autopolymerizing acrylic resin. The added resin will seal any gap in the region of the post dam and may even provide enough extra bulk to resist flexing.

Remaining teeth

When a few natural teeth remain but not enough or in sufficiently good condition to warrant their preservation, three plans of treatment are possible. They can be extracted and an immediate denture provided. They can be retained temporarily and added a few at a time to a transitional denture until a complete denture is made, or the roots of teeth can be retained as overdenture abutments. In selected cases it may even be possible to inhibit alveolar resorption by replacing the roots of unsaveable teeth with a biocompatible substitute like hydroxy-apatite.

Often the deciding factor is the patient's age. For a relatively young patient (below the age of 50) with neglected teeth (nowadays a much more rare occurrence) the obvious action is to provide an immediate denture. Techniques for immediate replacement of teeth are well documented and need no further amplification here. The young patient will adapt well to the changes involved and often prefers, especially if in full-time employment, to have treatment concentrated in this way into a few visits. Problems only occur when after insertion of the dentures the intervals for review are to be decided. Recall at 1 day and 1 week are mandatory and are needed to treat acute symptoms or to remove sutures and review healing. In the following weeks and months further review visits are needed to restore support and function to the denture as resorption progresses.

Even with the most careful system of review, the great changes in the orofacial region caused by provision of immediate dentures strain patients' powers of adaptation, and the treatment is best suited to the young or at least the physiologically young. Older patients adapt less well to tooth loss and for them it might be preferable to retain periodontally involved teeth as long as possible, despite loss of a little more alveolar bone, to prolong the period of adaptation. For such a person the transitional denture is intended.

The transitional partial denture is an excellent means of introducing elderly patients to complete dentures slowly and at a rate to which they can successfully adapt. Patients will often have preserved the remnants of their teeth without needing a partial denture, and only attend when the recent loss of a strategic tooth or teeth has caused an objectionable interference with function or appearance. If examination reveals that the remaining teeth are unsaveable or likely to be lost in the near future, an acrylic resin partial denture is made first and the patient allowed a prolonged period in which to adapt to its use. Adaptation is better if the denture base is designed to contact the lingual surfaces of the remaining teeth which can provide frictional support. For a conventional denture such a design would be discouraged on the grounds of hygiene, but it is unobjectionable for a transitional denture because the treatment plan involves loss of the remaining teeth, and contact of the denture with the lingual surfaces of the remaining teeth simplifies their addition when in the end it becomes necessary.

When the patient has adapted completely to the partial denture the remaining teeth are added a small number at a time. With elderly patients no surgical reduction of associated undercuts is performed. Instead, to improve stability, a labial or buccal flange is added a little at a time as resorption progresses. Gradually over a period of as long as several years the partial denture is converted to a complete denture by additions of autopolymerizing acrylic resin. Finally, the complete denture is replaced by one of less porous heat-cured resin which will maintain a permanently good appearance.

The disadvantage of the transitional denture is the large number of visits required. However, when patient adaptation is judged to be poor there is little alternative. Fortunately it usually takes place at a time of life when the patient has retired from full time employment and the numerous visits can be planned so that they do not interfere with the patient's leisure pursuits.

A case can sometimes be made for preserving the remaining teeth in a modified

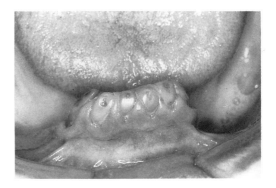

Fig. 1.22 Retention of six mandibular anterior roots has allowed the preservation of valuable alveolar bone in an otherwise atrophic jaw.

form. Preserving the roots of teeth enhances denture stability in several ways. Alveolar bone is retained which would otherwise be lost along with the denture stability afforded by a well developed alveolar process, and support is provided against the forces of mastication via the root faces (Fig. 1.22). Another equally important point is that a psychological reassurance is given to the patient that all is not yet lost. Preservation of proprioceptive sensation from the retained periodontal membranes is a debatable advantage.

Overdentures are becoming increasingly popular. Their provision is undoubtedly less traumatic, and it is usually preferable on health grounds for an elderly person to have the crown of an unrestorable tooth removed and the root retained than to endure the often prolonged experience of extraction, followed by frequent visits to preserve the stability of a denture whose support is resorbing rapidly. Further, removal of the crown of a mobile tooth will stabilize the root by improving the crown/root ratio and allow an otherwise valueless remnant to fulfil a useful supportive role.

Classically, complete overdentures are of three types, immediate, transitional and replacement, and while techniques are fairly standard there are controversial aspects. An immediate overdenture is analogous to a conventional complete immediate denture. Following any necessary endodontic treatment a denture is made precisely in the way of a conventional immediate denture. After the try-in stage, the teeth on the model which have been selected as overdenture abutments are cut down to just above the gingival margin before finishing the denture as normal. At the next visit the teeth which are to act as abutments are cut down to a low domed shape, the periphery of the dome being level with the gingival margin, and the endodontic access cavities sealed with amalgam. The fitting surface of the denture is then modified to fit accurately over the prepared abutments, first reducing high spots with the aid of disclosing wax and then restoring functional contact with autopolymerizing acrylic resin.

A transitional overdenture is analogous to a transitional partial denture. First a partial denture is made, then instead of the remaining teeth being extracted and added to the denture, they are root treated and converted into overdenture abutments, first reducing them to 1 mm or so above the gingival margin for the addition impression, then to the final form prior to the fit and final adjustment. Like the conventional transitional denture the technique is ideal for a patient who it is suspected will tolerate changes badly. Not only is surgical interference avoided but time is allowed for habituation to wearing a complete denture. When the only remaining teeth are elongated mandibular canines a transitional overdenture is easier than the complete immediate type. Fracture of the models frequently occurs at the cervical margins of the two remaining teeth when making an immediate denture and model trim-

ming is correspondingly more difficult to perform accurately.

A permanent overdenture is one constructed later when the prognosis for the immediate or transitional overdenture is assured. Because retained roots preserve a considerable mass of alveolus, part of which may form an undercut, a strengthener is usually added to the design to prevent fracture. To ensure correct functional loading a space is provided between the root surfaces and the metal base, and the metal casting is spaced from the root surfaces by an appropriately thick layer of foil prior to processing.

The subject of overdentures has been thoroughly covered of late[36] but some aspects of diagnosis can cause interesting problems. On purely functional grounds the first question to be answered before providing an overdenture is whether retention of the roots of the teeth is necessary. In other words, has the loss of teeth elsewhere in the mouth resulted in excess alveolar resorption? If areas elsewhere in the mouth do not show excessive alveolar bone loss after several years tooth loss and an adequate ridge form remains, it is questionable whether the extra expense of an overdenture is justified. This further implies that as resorption is a more prominent feature following mandibular tooth loss than maxillary tooth loss, overdenture therapy can be more easily justified in the mandible than the maxilla. Nevertheless, no matter which jaw is being treated, if any increase in face height is being contemplated, the extra support given by retained tooth roots is an advantage not to be discarded lightly.

Next it has to be decided whether the remaining teeth are suitable in site and form for preservation. If the root canal form is complex or if caries has destroyed much of the crown of the tooth to below the cervical margin, provision of an

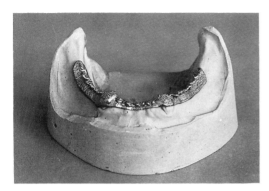

Fig. 1.23 Cast cobalt/chromium strengthener for a mandibular complete overdenture.

overdenture may be contraindicated on the grounds of difficulty in preserving the teeth. Nevertheless no matter how complex the root anatomy if, on a radiograph, obliteration of the canal is seen to have progressed to a marked extent in an elderly person, root canal therapy may well be unnecessary and removal of the crown will not endanger the pulp.

Mandibular canines are often the only teeth remaining when overdentures are planned. Their well known resistance to caries and massive root form ensure that they are the last to succumb to normal dental diseases. While their root size also makes them particularly suitable for denture support they are not ideal. Endodontic therapy can be difficult because they commonly have a complex root canal shape, and there is often a labial alveolar undercut which acts to weaken the denture, lessen physical retention and if large make for poor aesthetics. Extra cost may also be involved. If canines are preserved, the substantial amount of retained alveolar bone weakens the denture locally and adequate strength can often only be achieved by incorporating a metal strengthener, usually in the form of a cast metal base joining the exposed roots and extending for 2–3 cm towards the molar region (Fig.

1.23). On the grounds of ease of treatment more suitable mandibular teeth are incisors, and if possible premolars, neither of which are usually associated with large undercuts. Where a choice is possible a quadrilateral or tripod of support should be sought, with surplus teeth being extracted beforehand and added to an existing denture.

The final factor to be considered is the patient's state of oral hygiene. Caries will progress rapidly in the protected area of stagnation beneath a denture, and unless caries is controlled it will be found that overdentures have a limited life. Even when caries is judged to be unlikely it is important to emphasize oral hygiene procedures and to ensure that some form of caries prevention regime is followed. This can involve regular review by a hygienist for assessment and reinforcement of oral hygiene, and application of an anti-caries fluoride varnish to the exposed root surfaces. Anti-caries treatment can be provided at home by prescription of a supply of acidulated phosphate-buffered fluoride gel. A single drop can be placed by the patient on that part of the denture in contact with the root abutments each week. Alternatively, a small amount of a fluoridated dentifrice can be used daily.

It is sometimes best to retain roots to support an overdenture even when it is thought that their loss due to caries will be inevitable. The elderly habituate slowly to oral changes and only a long period of slow modification is well tolerated. An acceptable rate of progression is more likely with overdenture therapy and even though the abutment teeth will ultimately be lost, their preservation for a few more years allows the patient to become accustomed to a stable complete denture before the problems of post-extraction resorption are encountered. A conventional immediate denture means the

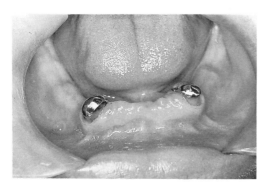

Fig. 1.24 Cast gold diaphragms have been present for 10 years in a patient with good oral hygiene. While the diaphragms have protected the occlusal surfaces, cervical toothbrush abrasion has occurred.

patient attempting to habituate simultaneously to the physical bulk of a denture while resorption is causing it to become progressively more unstable.

Cast metal diaphragms covering the exposed root surfaces are recommended by some clincians. Orginally they were reputed to have the advantage of preventing caries but this has been disputed recently,[37] and it is difficult to imagine how if oral hygiene is poor the presence of a metal diaphragm will do other than modify the site at which further caries occurs—if oral hygiene is poor there will be further loss of epithelial attachment with caries of the exposed cervical margins. The other claimed advantage is to reduce the amount of root surface abrasion caused by contact with a metal strengthener (Fig. 1.24). This intention is entirely laudable.

It is preferable that the root abutment shape for an immediate or transitional denture should be one which allows maximum strength of the denture base, and a low domed shape is to be preferred on the grounds that there is a thicker, stronger mass of acrylic. A permanent overdenture, however, may have a cast metal strengthener. Metal diaphragms

over the root faces then allow the operator to contour the abutment to any desired shape while not decreasing the strength of the denture base. A highly domed diaphragm can be incorporated with the resulting advantage of increased lateral stability.

Researchers in the field of complete denture prosthodontics have long searched for a means of inhibiting the avleolar resorption which follows extraction of unsaveable teeth. A recently developed technique aims to replace the lost root with a non-resorbable, biocompatible, tooth substitute which integrates with the remaining alveolar bone.[38] The first effective tooth root substitutes were cones of dense hydroxyapatite which were placed in sockets immediately after extraction. The only requirements from the patient, apart from good general health, are that at least 3 mm of tooth socket are available for implantation of the replicas. Proprietary kits of root replicas contain stainless steel socket gauges to assess the tooth and socket size after extraction, and matched hydroxyapatite cones which can be cut to the correct length and inserted firmly into the socket at least 2 mm below the alveolar crest.

While the method does appear to retain alveolar bone,[39] a proportion of root replicas exfoliate or are otherwise lost and patient confidence in the final outcome can diminish. One investigation showed that the proportion lost soon after implantation was approximately 12% and postulated that because the root replica most frequently lost was the canine (a tooth with a very variable root anatomy), the technique would always involve a high rate of loss unless more accurately fitting replicas could be manufactured.[40] A further proportion of replicas come to the surface at a later stage and while retaining their bony attachment are a source of annoyance to the

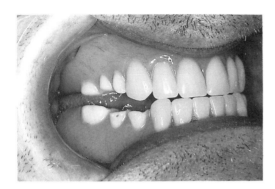

Fig. 1.25 Abnormal wear of posterior teeth due to the habitual chewing of boiled sweets.

patient. Such replicas can either be removed surgically if they irritate the patient, or the superficial portion can be reduced with a diamond bur to below the gingival margin and the mucosa allowed to cover it over once more.

Root replica implantation has been shown to preserve the alveolus but because of the problems of patient selection and post-insertion loss of replicas, the alternative procedure of filling extraction sockets with dense hydroxyapatite particles has been suggested.[41] This has the advantage of extreme simplicity. However, no physical restraint is placed on the particles which lie loose in the socket and inevitably many are lost in the immediate post-operative and healing phases, even when the patient is cautioned to avoid rinsing and use careful oral hygiene measures. Another disadvantage is the cost. Root replica implants are relatively cheap and the equivalent amount of dense hydroxyapatite particles more expensive by a factor of 10 or 20.

The denture

Any available dentures are now examined. If worn satisfactorily they are a valuable source of information and record the spatial relationships of teeth and base which the patient tolerates. Apart from using them in duplication and denture copying procedures, provided their fit is still reasonable, a record of the fitting surfaces in silicone putty can be taken at this stage and this will provide a model for making special trays or even registration blocks (see Appendix I).

The presence of plaque and food debris on dentures indicates poor oral hygiene which in turn implies a tendency to infection by candidal organisms. Before embarking on prosthodontic treatment the presence of plaque should be confirmed to the patient by use of disclosing solution and a warning given that oral health can only be maintained by good denture cleansing, a warning that is especially relevant if an overdenture is anticipated. A review of the methods of denture hygiene is given in Chapter 8.

Any wear or discolouration should also be noted. Wear of the occlusal surfaces of dentures is to be expected and should be in proportion to their age. Acrylic teeth wear to a far greater extent than porcelain. Sometimes wear is concentrated at one point of the occlusal surface posteriorly and is the consequence of habitual chewing of some food item—usually hard sweets (Fig. 1.25). Extreme localized wear of the incisal edge to produce an area where no incisal contact occurs is typical of a pipe smoker. To ensure that a pipe smoker can both smoke and wear his dentures comfortably the pattern of attrition may have to be reproduced in the new dentures or the mouthpiece of the pipe warmed and bent so that, pivoting on the mandibular anteriors, it gives support to the maxillary denture (Fig. 1.26). Where differential wear (or modification of the positions of the teeth to give an arrangement similar to differential wear) is associated with the embouchure of a musical instrument the

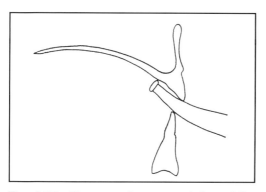

Fig. 1.26 Diagrammatic representation of the bend to be put in a pipe stem if a smoker encounters difficulties with stability of the maxillary denture.

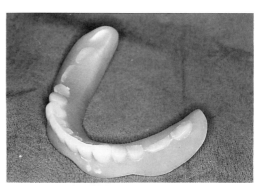

Fig. 1.27 Extreme general tooth wear caused by involuntary grinding movements in a case of tardive dyskinesia.

arrangement has usually been established by the previous dentist and will have to be incorporated also in the new. There is little chance that the need will be missed even after the most cursory assessment. Players of wind instruments who require a particular tooth position are always concerned to bring this to the attention of the operator and will explain in detail the required modifications. Abnormal patterns of occlusal wear are encountered in some elderly patients as a consequence of tardive dyskinesia which results from therapy with antipsychotic drugs (Fig. 1.27).[42] It is immediately confirmed by the associated uncontrollable chewing or grimacing movements. Apart from ensuring that dentures are as trauma free as possible, there is little that the prosthodontist can do.

When the wear involves the polished surface, some form of abnormal denture cleansing routine should be suspected and the patient warned against the use of agents other than those specifically formulated for denture wearers, although if the patient prefers to use conventional toothpaste little damage will be done. If the fitting surface of a recently constructed denture is found to be smooth but ill fitting, it is likely that the patient

has been in the habit of adjusting the denture himself with an abrasive such as steel wool or an abrasive pad. A warning must be given that any future adjustments to a denture must only be made by the operator in the surgery.

Bleaching of dentures is not uncommon and can result when strong hypochlorite solutions are mistakenly used as part of the denture hygiene routine. Reputable denture cleansers will not cause damage or discolouration of denture base acrylic when used in normal concentrations and under the recommended conditions. Bleaching with proprietary cleansers will only result when an enthusiastic patient decides that the denture cleansing effect ought to be enhanced by increasing the concentration of the cleanser or employing it for prolonged periods of time at temperatures higher than those recommended in the instructions.

Micro-valves were once used by despairing clincians to provide retention for the dentures of patients when all attempts at conventional treatment had failed. For success they depended on forming a small relief chamber beneath the denture which was in turn connected to the polished surface via a tunnel furnished with a small one-way valve. Sucking on the

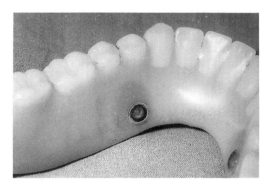

Fig. 1.28 In a final attempt to secure retention of a mandibular complete denture *two* micro-valves were inserted. Their failure was due to the common difficulty associated with mandibular complete dentures—ensuring adequate peripheral seal.

valve allowed the contents of the chamber to be evacuated into the mouth. The reduced pressure in the chamber aided retention of the denture. For its success the technique demanded creation of an effective peripheral seal and was normally reserved for maxillary dentures (Fig. 1.28). Even when successful the effect was temporary, being nullified by overgrowth of soft tissue into the chamber and blockage of the valve by food debris. Discovery of a micro-valve in a patient's denture is now an indication of possible difficulty ahead.

Some elderly, edentulous patients may have had the fitting surface of a mandibular denture lined with a semi-permanent soft liner. Two forms are available at present, a silicone rubber and a heat-cured plasticised poly(ethyl methacrylate) which softens at mouth temperatures. For maximum benefit the linings should be 3 mm thick. Neither are long lasting, although with care they survive up to 2 years. The problem with both types is adhesion and both tend to separate from the base, some after a very short period of time. The poly (ethyl methacrylate) types have the additional disadvantages that they discolour

easily. In order to improve adhesion of the lining to the base it is sometimes boxed in, but the boxed edge can be lost at the insertion stage if adjustments to the periphery are needed. Both types of lining are difficult to adjust and polish and special abrasive stones are needed for silicone rubber linings.

The ideal patient for such a lining is difficult to identify. There may be advantages in limiting their use to elderly patients with pain beneath their mandibular denture from a thin friable mucosa. Where pain is caused by irregular bony spicules or prominences which the patient is unwilling to have removed, semi-permanent soft liners are often provided in desperation, at the patient's request, when all else has failed. Most often they are provided because the previous denture has had such a lining and the patient is now addicted to it. Semi-permanent soft liners should never be provided when the mucosa is friable and associated with a lack of saliva. The increased friction merely makes the situation worse.

Finally, the dentures are examined in occlusion in the mouth. When a denture has been worn for a considerable time without modification the combined effects of occlusal wear and alveolar resorption cause a gradual reduction in the face height. In time a protrusive path of closure is adopted and when associated with incisal wear can cause a change in the overjet with a reversal of the normal incisal relations (Fig. 1.29). It is then difficult to record a consistent retruded contact position without the patient lapsing into a faulty habitual position. Many experienced clinicians advise that to aid the accurate recording of the jaw relations the face height is increased before new dentures are made, the purpose being to accustom the patient afresh to a normal occlusal face height and position the mandible in a more normal, retruded

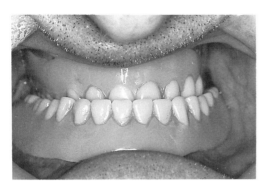

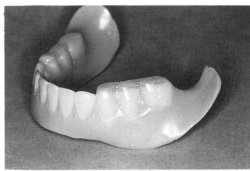

Fig. 1.29 Reversal of incisor relationship caused by occlusal wear and postural overclosure.

Fig. 1.30 The face height has been increased by clear autopolymerizing acrylic additions to the occlusal surfaces of the mandibular denture.

position. The difficulty lies in determining the extent to which an elderly patient can tolerate a return to a more normal occlusal face height.

Two techniques can be employed but with the proviso that modifications should be applied with caution. If well tolerated dentures are permanently modified and subsequently become uncomfortable, patient confidence will be immediately lost. Duplicate dentures, which can be modified with impunity, must be made if there is any doubt as to the patient's ability to adapt to the proposed changes.

The first technique for restoring lost face height involves providing autopolymerizing acrylic resin occlusal pivots in the premolar region.[43] A small amount of clear resin is mixed and placed bilaterally on the occlusal surface of the mandibular denture in the second premolar region and using a folded piece of aluminium foil as a matrix, formed into a trapezoid prism the flattened upper surface of which contacts the opposing denture on occlusion evenly at the increased face height. After removing the foil which has served to prevent adhesion with the maxillary denture and reduce intercuspal guidance, an even occlusal contact is provided in the premolar region allowing the mandible to retrude without causing interference or instability of the denture. If the patient can tolerate it, any further necessary increase in the height of the pivot can be made a few weeks later.

The technique of occlusal pivots is simple but patients may feel, unwarrantedly, that not enough occlusal contact is provided for effective chewing. An alternative which takes a little more time is to add a layer of clear autopolymerizing acrylic resin to the entire posterior occlusal surface of the mandibular denture, and providing even occlusal contact with the opposing denture by instructing the patient to close gently into the doughing mixture after smearing the opposing teeth with petroleum jelly. Once bilateral contact is made at an increased face height the denture is removed and placed in warm water for polymerization to be completed. The new occlusal surface is then adjusted to give a smooth surface without antero-posterior cuspal interferences (Fig. 1.30).

A history of fracture of the denture base should be an indication to search for the cause. Often the cause is impact, with the denture being dropped while being cleaned, and elderly patients are

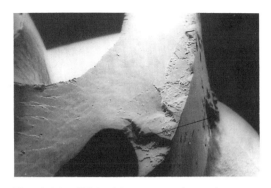

Fig. 1.31 SEM of fracture surface of a complete mandibular denture. The rough surface of crack initiation (arrowed) is related to a surface notch where a tooth has been lost due to inadequate adhesive bond.

particularly liable to break dentures in this way. If it is suspected that due to the patient's age or medical condition, fracture is going to be a recurrent problem and the tendency is not going to be overcome by instructions in denture care and cleansing, it is worthwhile recommending replacement of the denture by one made from an impact-resistant resin. Such resins consist of rubber/acrylic copolymers, the rubber particles within the matrix serving to inhibit crack propagation.

Other types of fracture are due to fatigue and the cause will be easily detected. The denture may be old and ill-fitting, when the mismatch between the fitting surface and the denture-bearing surface causes it to flex under the force of mastication. Alternatively, it may be new and provided for a patient with too little interalveolar space to allow enough bulk of acrylic for adequate strength. Thirdly, some form of stress concentrating factor may be present, for example a notch to provide relief for a fraenum, or the fracture may be initiated from the indentations in the resin resulting from using porcelain teeth, or acrylic teeth with a poor adhesive bond to the base (Fig. 1.31).[44] Under these circumstances repair

can only be a temporary expedient and the basic cause of the fracture must be eliminated. If it is impossible to eliminate the causative factor some form of strengthening must be used. Either a stronger resin must be used (e.g. polycarbonate), or a cast metal base must be incorporated. Impact resistant resins are not indicated.

Special tests

The number of special tests of major significance in complete denture prosthodontics is limited. First among these is radiographic assessment. All standing teeth should be assessed radiographically, a mandatory procedure for overdenture abutments. Radiographic assessment is also advisable for teeth which are to be extracted from an elderly person because conditions which will complicate extraction, such as hypercementosis, are more common. A radiographic scan of edentulous areas is recommended. Several investigators have shown that the incidence of residual pathology revealed in this way approaches 30%[45] and it could be negligent to omit radiography if the past medical or dental history reveals trauma to the jaws or a history of difficult extractions. If facilities are available, panoramic radiography is the method of choice.

Patients' symptoms may lead the operator to suspect allergy or hypersensivity to acrylic resin. In practice, some patients with painful dentures (or even their despairing dentists) have already made the tentative diagnosis of acrylic allergy. Most such cases of apparent allergy are due to infection or occlusal trauma and careful investigation will reveal the previously unsuspected cause. Cases of true allergy to poly (methyl methacrylate) are rare and are associated with soreness, reddening and desquamation of the mucosa in contact with the denture. Other symptoms which may be present and help to confirm the diagnosis are redness of the skin in contact with spectacle frames, and redness and itching associated with the wearing of certain articles of clothing, namely those containing acrylic fibre. When allergy is suspected and the symptoms cannot be related to infection or trauma, tests for allergy may be carried out after referral to a dermatologist. Contact tests involving application to the skin, with hypo-allergic tape, of small pieces of acrylic or scrapings of the denture are often used.[46] A lymphocyte transformation test will give a more precise result.[47]

When allergy to acrylic is confirmed the only solution is to provide a denture made from another material. Vulcanite is not the only alternative and dentures can be made of polycarbonate, which also has superior physical properties. Unfortunately the costs are substantially greater because polycarbonate requires an injection moulding process. While Nylon has been suggested in the past as an alternative denture base for cases of allergy, it is dimensionally unstable. In the mouth it absorbs water and expands, losing retention.

Although allergy to poly (methyl methacrylate) is rare, sensitivity to acrylic monomer is more common and may follow provision of a denture which has been insufficiently cured, resulting in a high proportion of residual monomer. Alternatively, autopolymerizing resin (which unless carefully cured contains large amounts of residual monomer)[48] may have been used as a repair or reline material. Replacement of the denture by one which has been properly processed is the obvious remedy. An alternative is to make the denture from a light-cured acrylic, the dough of which contains no monomer. The cost is greater (to reflect the greater technical costs involved), and discolouration occurs after a time due to slight porosity.

Two other forms of test may also be prescribed. Of these, the significance of bacteriological investigation in cases of denture stomatitis has already been discussed, and when dealing with the prosthodontic problems resulting from a dry mouth, saliva function tests are rarely of significance except in clinically obvious cases.

References

1. Bergendal, B. The relative importance of tooth loss and denture wearing in Swedish adults. *Comm Dent Health* **6**:103–111, 1989.
2. Collet, H. Influence of dentist–patient relationship on attitude and adjustment to dental treatment. *J Am Dent Assoc* **79**:879–884, 1969.
3. Kincey, J., Bradshaw, P. and Ley, P. Patients' satisfaction and reported acceptance of advice in general practice. *J R Col Gen Practit* **25**:558–562, 1975.
4. Davenport, J.C., and Heath, J.R. The copy denture technique. *Br Dent J* **155**:162–163, 1983.
5. Heath, J.R. and Basker, R.M. The dimensional variability of duplicate dentures produced in alginate investment. *Br Dent J* **144**:111–114, 1978.
6. Patterson, N. Musicians and dentures. *J Am Dent Assoc* **67**:862–864, 1963.
7. Porter, M.M. Dental problems in wind instrument playing. VI—single reed instruments—the embouchure denture. *Br Dent J* **124**:34–36, 1968.
8. Lamey, P.J. and Lewis M.A.O. Oral medicine in practice: burning mouth syndrome. *Br Dent J* **167**:197–200, 1989.
9. Ong, T.K., Lancer, J.M. and Brook, I.M. Inhalation of a denture fragment complicating facial trauma. *Br J Oral Maxillofac Surg* **26**:511–513, 1988.

10. McCord, J.F., Tyson, K.W. and Blair, I.S. A sectional complete denture for a patient with microstomia. *J Prosthet Dent* **61**:645–647, 1989.

11. Weisenfeld, D., Stewart, A.M. and Mason, D.K. A critical assessment of oral lubricants in patients with xerostomia. *Br Dent J* **155**:155–157, 1983.

12. Neill, D.J. and Glaysher, K.L. Identifying the denture space. *J Oral Rehabil* **9**:259–277, 1982.

13. Budtz-Jorgensen, E., Stenderup, A. and Grabowski, M. An epidemiological study of yeasts in elderly denture wearers. *Com Dent Oral Epidemiol* **3**:115–119, 1975.

14. Dorey, J.L., Blasberg, B., MacEntee, M.I. and Conklin, R.J. Oral mucosal disorders in denture wearers. *J Prosthet Dent* **53**:210–213, 1985.

15. Jenning, J.K. and MacDonald, D.J. Histological, microbiological and haematological investigations in denture-induced stomatitis. *J Dent* **18**:102–106, 1990.

16. Arendorf, T.M. and Walker, D.M. Denture stomatitis: a review. *J Oral Rehabil* **14**:217–227, 1987.

17. Arendorf, T.M. and Walker, D.M. Oral candidal populations in health and disease. *Br Dent J* **147**:267–272, 1979.

18. Lamb, D.J. and Douglas, C.W.I. Treatment of denture stomatitis by a sustained drug-delivery device, a preliminary study. *J Dent* **16**:219–221, 1988.

19. Douglas, C.W.I and Lamb, D.J. Denture sonication as a means of assessing denture-associated candidosis. *Gerodontics* **4**:289–292, 1988.

20. Shen, K and Gongloff, R.K. Prevalence of 'combination syndrome' among denture patients. *J Prosthet Dent* **62**:642–644, 1989.

21. Kent, J.N., Finger, I.M., Quinn, J.H. and Guerra, L.R. Hydroxylapatite ridge reconstruction: clinical experiences, complications and technical modifications. *J Oral Maxillofac Surg* **44**:37–49, 1986.

22. Frame, J.W. Hydroxyapatite as a biomaterial for alveolar ridge augmentation. *Int J Oral Maxillofac Surg* **16**:642–655, 1987.

23. Brook, I.M., Craig, G.T., Douglas, C.W.I. et al. Management of the mobile fibrous ridge in the atrophic maxilla. *Br Dent J* (Letter) **162**:413, 1987.

24. Mehlisch, D.R., Taylor, T.D., Leibold, D.G. et al. Evaluation of collagen/hydroxyapatite for augmenting deficient alveolar ridges: a preliminary study. *J Oral Maxillofac Surg* **45**:408–413, 1987.

25. Tallgren, A. The continuing reduction of the residual alveolar ridges in complete denture wearers: a mixed longitudinal study covering 25 years. *J Prosthet Dent* **27**:120–132, 1972.

26. Kalk, W. and de Baat, C. Some factors connected with alveolar bone resorption. *J Dent* **17**:162–165, 1989.

27. Berg, E. A 2-year follow-up study of patient satisfaction with new complete dentures. *J Dent* **16**:160–165, 1988.

28. Kent, J.N. Reconstruction of the edentulous alveolar ridge with hydroxyapatite. *Dent Clin N Am* **30**(2):231–257, 1986.

29. Brook, I.M. and Lamb, D.J. Two stage combined vestibuloplasty and partial mandibular augmentation with hydroxyapatite. *J Oral Maxillofac Surg* **47**:331–335, 1989.

30. Branemark, P.I. Osseointegration and its experimental background. *J Prosthet Dent* **50**:399–410, 1983.

31. Ellis, B., Lamb, D.J. and McDonald, P. A study of the composition and diffusion characteristics of a soft liner. *J Dent* **7**:133–140, 1979.

32. Davenport, J.C., Wilson, H.J. and Basker, R.M. The compatibility of tissue conditioners with denture cleansers and chlorhexidine. *J. Dent* **6**:239–246, 1978.

33. Brook, I.M. and Lamb, D.J. Treatment of denture-induced hyperplasia. *Dental Update* **14**:288–295, 1987.

34. McCartney, J.W. Flange adaptation discrepancy, palatal base distortion and induced malocclusion caused by processing acrylic resin maxillary complete dentures. *J Prosthet Dent* **52**:545–553, 1984.

35. Morris, J.C., Khan, Z. and von Fraunhofer, J.A. Palatal shape and flexural strength of maxillary denture bases. *J Prosthet Dent* **53**:670–673, 1985.

36. Basker, R.M., Harrison, A. and Ralph, J.P. Overdentures in general dental prac-

tice. London: BDA Publications, 1988.

37. Ettinger, R.L., Taylor, T.D. and Scandrett, F.R. Treatment needs of overdenture patients in a longitudinal study: five-year results. *J Prosthet Dent* **52**:532–537, 1984.

38. Quinn, J.H., Kent J.N., Hunter, R.G. and Schaffer, C.M. Preservation of the alveolar ridge with hydroxylapatite tooth root substitutes. *J Am Dent Assoc* **110**:189–193, 1985.

39. Sattayasanskul, W., Brook, I.M. and Lamb, D.J. Dense hydroxyapatite root replica implantation: measurement of alveolar ridge preservation. *Int J Oral Maxillofac Imp* **3**:203–207, 1988.

40. Brook, I.M., Sattayasanskul, W. and Lamb, D.J. Dense hydroxyapatite root replica implantation: tooth site and success rate. *Br Dent J* **164**:212–215, 1988.

41. Bell, D.H. Particle versus solid forms of hydroxyapatite as a treatment modality to preserve residual alveolar ridges. *J Prosthet Dent* **56**:322–326, 1986.

42. Langer, A. Chemopsychotherapy and its role in prosthetic failures in elderly patients. *J Prosthet Dent* **52**:14–19, 1984.

43. Watt, D.M., and Lindsay, K.N. Occlusal pivot appliances. *Br Dent J* **132**:110–112, 1972.

44. Lamb, D.J., Ellis, B. and van Noort, R. The fracture topography of acrylic dentures fractured in service. *Biomaterials* **6**:110–112, 1985.

45. Keur, J.J., Campbell, J.P.S., McCarthy, J.F. and Ralph, W.J. Radiological findings in 1135 patients. *J Oral Rehabil* **14**:183–191, 1987.

46. Lamey, P.J. and Lewis, M.A.O. Oral medicine in practice: orofacial allergic reactions. *Br Dent J* **168**:59–63, 1990.

47. Devlin, H. and Watts, D.C. Acrylic "allergy". *Br Dent J* **157**:272–275, 1984.

48. Lamb, D.J., Ellis, B. and Priestly, D. The effect of process variables on levels of residual monomer in autopolymerizing acrylic resin. *J Dent* **11**:80–88, 1983.

Chapter 2

Impression Stage

Most practitioners have favourite impression materials and techniques. An experienced operator will have developed considerable manipulative skill when using them and produce good results in a variety of difficult clinical situations. Such skill is invaluable and this section does not aim to change any practitioner's basic technique, but instead seeks to provide a rational criticism of existing methods, summarize the problems which can arise, and introduce for consideration some techniques which can be applied to those patients with special needs.

Functional anatomy of impressions

Primary impressions

Impressions for complete dentures are conventionally made in two stages. The primary impression records the useful anatomy of the edentulous mouth so that a model can be cast on which an accurately fitting special tray can be made. An impression material is usually chosen which is viscous enough to displace unsupported tissues and ensure that all relevant anatomy is recorded, including the retromolar pad and the junction of hard and soft palate. In doing so it also

distends the sulcus slightly beyond its functional extent, which makes the impression unsuitable for the purpose of casting a working model.

To be certain that the mandibular primary impression is adequate it must record the entire lingual and buccal sulci, including the external oblique ridges, the entire retromolar pads, and any lingual or buccal fraenal attachments. The maxillary primary impression must similarly record the sulcus in its entirety, including the hamular or pterygo-maxillary notches, any fraenal attachments, and the soft palate as far back as the palatal foveae. In the absence of well defined palatal foveae, the palatal extension should reach an imaginary line joining the hamular notches.

When making primary impressions efforts should be made to limit the overextension which results from the need to employ an impression material of relatively high viscosity. Inevitably, the impressions are made by an open-mouth technique and with the mouth maintained open the facial muscles, which in function would restrict buccal and labial extension of the impression, are lax and easily displaced. At the same time the muscles of floor of the mouth are engaged in maintaining the open-mouth position, the hyoid bone is depressed and the mandibular lingual sulcus is deeper

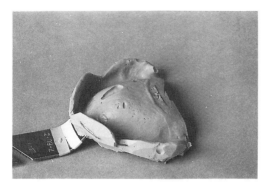

Fig. 2.1A A preliminary alginate impression trimmed back with a scalpel to the depth of the sulcus and junction of hard and soft palate. The fraenal attachments have also been relieved.

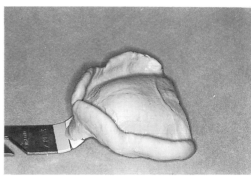

Fig. 2.1.B To complete the impression a wash is taken in a more fluid mix of alginate.

than would be encountered in normal oral function.

As a general method, to limit over-extension and simulate functional activity of the relevant muscles while taking primary impressions, muscle trimming is carried out. With the tray seated in the mouth but before the impression material has set, traction on the surrounding muscles may be exerted via the modiolus. For both the mandibular and maxillary impressions the modiolus is drawn inward and forward to determine the functional buccal sulcus. For the labial sulcus the modiolus is drawn backwards and inwards and supplemented by downwards and inwards pressure on the upper lip and upwards and inwards pressure on the lower lip. A reasonable functional representation of the mandibular lingual sulcus is achieved by protruding the tongue.

Primary impressions in irreversible hydrocolloid (alginate) can be trimmed back to the appropriate anatomical landmarks using a technique similar to that advised by Halperin et al.[1] This involves cutting the mandibular impression material arbitrarily back to the distal edge of the retromolar pad, the external oblique ridge and the deepest part of the labial and lingual sulci. For a better resolution

of the periphery the fraenal attachments are relieved before a wash impression is made in a fluid mix of material and associated with further muscle trimming. The maxillary impression is treated in an analogous way, reducing and thinning the extensions into the sulcus (Fig. 2.1A and B).

Working impressions

Special, or custom trays allow an impression to be made which is an accurate record of the functional denture-bearing area. By adjusting the tray accurately to the functional periphery and by using a fluid impression material an accurate working model can be cast. Because the periphery of the second or working impression is determined principally by tissues in their functional position rather than as displaced by the impression material, its extent is less than that of the primary impression.

In addition to the residual alveolar ridge, a mandibular working impression should record the reflection of the sulcus as determined by the insertions and movements of the surrounding muscles. Fraenal attachments must not be distorted by unrelieved special trays. Pos-

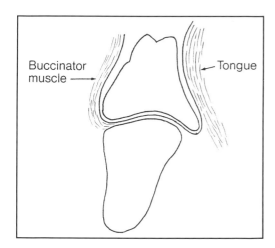

Fig. 2.2 A diagram of the lingual periphery of a mandibular denture extended into the retromylohyoid region, serving to promote stability by supporting the tongue.

teriorly the impression should not extend beyond the retromolar pad, otherwise in this region the future denture will be supported by unattached mucosa and will either be displaced by the underlying musculature or, if the denture is well retained, traumatize the mucosa. Controversy exists over whether to extend the impression lingually in the molar region beyond the mylohyoid attachment and into the retromylohyoid fossa. It is easier to end the impression at the mylohyoid ridge. Ending here ensures that there will be no lingual extension to be displaced, either by the mylohyoid muscle in the molar region, or by the floor of the mouth if the lingual extension extends distally beyond the mylohyoid attachment. Some patients permit functional lingual extensions to be made beyond the mylohyoid ridge into the retromylohyoid fossa and thereby gain additional stability for their denture, the extension being supported and stabilized by the base of the tongue (Fig. 2.2).

Like the mandibular impression, the maxillary impression records the undis-

torted reflection of the entire periphery along with any fraenal attachments. While the hamular notches must be recorded it is unnecessary to record distally far beyond the functional limit represented by the palpable junction of hard and soft palate.

Apart from incomplete extension, working impressions may show a number of faults. The commonest is a defect in the deepest part of the sulcus. Some materials, for example zinc oxide/eugenol impression paste, allow additions to be made in the same material, taking care to judge accurately the extra quantity of material required and by ensuring that the impression is completely reseated, not allowing any extra paste to flow onto the fitting surface. Other impression materials are more difficult to correct. If defects are small and "pedunculated", they can either be filled with soft wax or remain on the impression and be removed from the model. Never replace extensive sections of the periphery with soft disclosing-type wax. It distorts when the model is cast.

Penetration of the impression tray through the impression material is another common fault and causes the tissue in contact with the tray to be forcibly adapted to its shape. The impression must be repeated or alternatively, if the surface to be recorded is not undercut, a wash can be taken.

Another fault is one which is commonest when using irreversible hydrocolloids. Alginate is a popular impression material but does not adhere to the tray without help. Debonding is common despite putting perforations in the tray to mechanically lock the material in place and applying a tray adhesive. Always examine impressions carefully to ensure that debonding has not occurred. It is especially frequent in the post dam region and it is advisable to cut away any

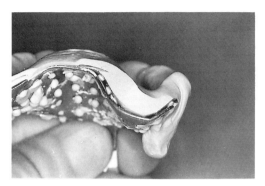

Fig. 2.3 Impression material has detached from the tray and the defect is revealed after cutting back the material in the post dam region.

surplus set impression material extending over the soft palate in order to examine the interface between impression material and tray (Fig. 2.3). Unless the bond is intact the resulting model will be inaccurate.

Denture retention

In textbooks the amount of stress laid on making accurate impressions highlights the importance of a close fit between the denture and its supporting tissues which in its turn is responsible for good retention. Retention may be defined as the ability of a denture at rest to resist forces displacing it at right angles away from the denture-bearing surface and for a complete denture is a function of the physical properties of saliva. Analogies are usually drawn between the clinical situation and two circular parallel plates separated by a liquid (Fig. 2.4). Under these conditions Stephan's law can be applied[2] and the force (F) necessary to increase the separation of the plates expressed as:

$$F = 3/4. \, \eta A^2/t. \, (1/h_1{}^2 - 1/h_2{}^2) \qquad (1)$$

Where η = the viscosity of the liquid

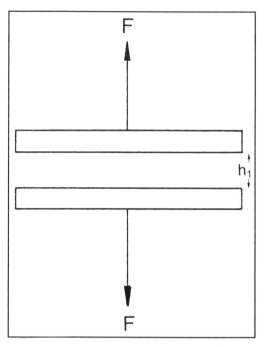

Fig. 2.4. Two circular parallel plates of area A, initial distance apart h_1, surrounded by a fluid medium of viscosity η, and being separated by force F.

A = the area of the plate
t = the time of force application
h_1 = initial plate separation
h_2 = final plate separation

If h_2 is much larger than h_1 the equation can be simplified to:

$$F = 3/4. \, \eta A^2/t. \, 1/h_1{}^2 \qquad (2)$$

The relationship expressed in equation (2) shows that the force required to displace a denture is proportional to the viscosity of the saliva fluid film and the square of the area of the denture, and inversely proportional to the square of the initial distance separating the denture from the supporting tissues and the time of force application.

The relationship allows a number of clinical inferences to be made. Obviously the degree of retention possessed by a denture depends critically on the area of its fitting surface and hence the requirement to extend the denture base to the maximum allowed by muscle insertions. While the degree of closeness of fit is also of great significance, the degree of irregularity of the fitting surface does not appear to be important, because the relevant area has been shown to be that projected onto a plane at right angles to the direction of movement.[3]

Retention of a denture is also affected by the viscosity of saliva and the greater the viscosity of saliva the better the retention. This principle is utilized by pharmaceutical companies in the preparation of denture adhesives. If a suitable polymer (usually polyethylene oxide or carboxymethyl cellulose), is applied to the fitting surface of a denture it will dissolve in saliva to produce solutions with viscosities of the order of 10^6 poise and substantially improve denture retention.[4] Even without such artificial aids saliva has properties which increase its viscosity above that of water. The glycoproteins and proteoglycans dissolved in saliva not only increase the viscosity but provide it with pseudoplastic properties. In other words, at the low shear rates encountered in the mouth when mastication is not taking place, saliva acts as a semi-solid.

As mentioned above, the force required to displace a complete denture is inversely proportional to the square of the distance which separates it from the denture-bearing area. To a considerable extent the accuracy with which the impression has been recorded will determine denture retention by establishing a close fit between the two surfaces. This is the justification for the practice (amply confirmed on the clinic) of increasing denture retention by improving the closeness of fit at the periphery and so selectively decreasing the initial distance of separation (h_1) at crucial sites. Obvious examples are the post dam on maxillary dentures and the success, in terms of retention, of techniques designed to cause an impression material to record the tissues of the periphery under increased pressure.

Although complete dentures will resist large displacing forces of brief duration, Stephan's law implies that a denture will be displaced by even a small force if it is applied for a long enough time. This is a well recognized clinical problem. With experience, patients learn to reposition their complete dentures involuntarily when speaking for prolonged periods and the main reason for providing balanced articulation is to prevent such reflex movements acting to displace the denture by a leverage effect, when they are applied other than in the intercuspal position.

Equations (1) and (2) are valid if we assume that the circular parallel plates are completely immersed in liquid. In the mouth, the dentures are not necessarily completely immersed in saliva all of the time, hence a meniscus can form at the periphery and surface tension can be included among the factors which enhance retention. If a capillary film exists between two circular parallel plates such that a meniscus forms at the edge, then the pressure inside the film is less than that outside the film. The difference in pressure is given by the Laplace formula (Fig. 2.5):[5]

$$p'' - p' = \sigma \left(1/r_1 - 1/r_2 \right) \qquad (3)$$

Where p'' = pressure on the concave side

    p' = pressure on the convex side

    r_1 = one principal radius of curvature of the film

    r_2 = other principal radius of curvature of the film

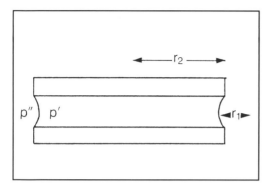

Fig. 2.5 Two circular parallel plates separated by a fluid film of surface tension σ. Principal radii of curvature are r_1 and r_2, pressures on convex and concave sides are p' and p'', respectively.

$$\sigma = \text{surface tension of the liquid}$$

The relationship has been adapted by Barbenel[3] to express the difference between the pressure in a saliva film separating a complete denture from its supporting tissues and the pressure in the mouth (i.e. atmospheric pressure). Under these circumstances:

$$p = 2T/h \qquad (4)$$

Where p = the reduction in pressure inside the film

T = the surface tension of saliva

h = the distance between the denture and its supporting tissues

Investigators have debated the influence of salivary surface tension on the retention of complete dentures and its importance now appears less than was once thought. Any positive effect that surface tension has must depend on there being an intact saliva/air interface at the periphery of the denture, a condition which could exist only during speech,

when it would be extremely advantageous. At rest with the lips in contact and the intra-oral space occluded, or when eating or drinking, the integrity of any peripheral saliva/air interface would be destroyed and the effect of surface tension would become negligible. Nevertheless, it may have a significant effect at critical times and the possible beneficial effect when speaking cannot be disproved. Any effect would be enhanced by a close fit between the denture and the denture-bearing tissues (h), again emphasizing the importance of accurate impression techniques.

It has been claimed in the past that the wettability of the denture base by saliva can be significant in denture retention,[6] saliva being regarded as an adhesive and its intimate contact with the adherend being ensured by good wettability of the denture base. Wettability can be expressed as being inversely proportional to the equilibrium contact angle, which in turn is related to the surface tensions or surface energies of the materials concerned by the "Young" equation:

$$\gamma_{sv} - \gamma_{sl} = \gamma_{lv} \cdot \cos\theta \qquad (5)$$

Where θ = equilibrium contact angle

γ_{sv} = surface tension or surface energy of the solid/vapour interface

g_{sl} = surface tension or surface energy of the solid/liquid interface

γ_{lv} = surface tension or surface energy of the liquid/vapour interface

Attempts have been made in the past to improve denture retention by either enhancing the wettability of acrylic by coating its surface with fine silica particles,[7] or alternatively by using a water absorbing acrylic.[8] However, results were recorded without taking into account the time dependent nature of retention by a fluid film. In any case, even if the bond between saliva and the denture base could be improved by these means, denture retention would still be limited by shearing of the saliva film under stress.

Earlier sources claim that atmospheric pressure is involved in complete denture retention. Undoubtedly, when surrounded by a concave meniscus, pressure inside the fluid film between the denture and the denture-bearing surface is less than that in the mouth, which is presumably near to atmospheric. This is not to imply that atmospheric pressure in itself has any role to play in retention. There are no reliable reports of altered denture retention when in aeroplanes or pressure chambers! In any case, even if differences were encountered it would be difficult to prove that they were due to alterations in atmospheric pressure and not a consequence of changes mediated by the autonomic nervous system.

Impression techniques

As patients have come to expect a higher quality prosthodontic service, so sophisticated impression techniques have been developed to enhance retention and stability. While the various techniques have been advocated by their originators with great enthusiasm, individual claims for success have been mostly based on clinical experience and none have had their long-term superiority proved by clinical trial based on the criterion of patient satisfaction. Until valid clinical trials have been reported it will be best to view the various methods as adjuncts to one's basic technique and judge their quality not just on their theoretical merits, or on satisfactory final results achieved in individual cases, but by the ease with which

they can be adopted and the ease with which they allow production of high quality impressions. In considering the more popular techniques it is easiest to classify them according to whether they attempt to improve either retention or stability.

Techniques to improve retention

Closed/open mouth technique

The greatest tests of denture retention occur when a patient is eating or speaking. When eating, the mouth is closed, and when speaking the mouth is still not opened to the extent corresponding to the degree of opening occurring during open-mouth impression making. If at the various degress of mouth opening the sulcus varies in depth, closed-mouth impressions should provide greatest overall retention because the denture periphery accurately fits the sulcus at the time of greatest need. Further, it is known that on opening and closing the mouth, slight medial and lateral elastic strain of the body of the mandible takes place under the influence of the medial and lateral resultant forces produced by the muscles of mastication. Theoretically, therefore, if the mandibular impression is recorded by a closed-mouth technique at the face height of the future denture, the denture will be an accurate fit during mastication. It is by such rationalizations that closed-mouth techniques claim an advantage over the normal open-mouth techniques.

With closed-mouth impressions, the working impressions are made at the registration stage to ensure that they are made at the correct face height—and also to avoid the necessity for another visit. Consequently, the record blocks have to be based in a relatively rigid material like acrylic or shellac. By recording the working impressions in the record blocks the extra final thickness of impression material will increase the ultimate face height by a significant amount. Hence, when recording the face height the occlusal face height established by the rims should be 1 or 2 mm less than the final face height required.

When a closed-mouth impression technique is used, even contact of the prepared blocks is first established in the retruded contact position at the slightly reduced face height that is recommended. After coating the bases of the blocks with the impression material they are reseated in the mouth and the patient encouraged to close again in the retruded contact position. To reproduce normal movements of the muscles surrounding the sulcus the patient can be given a small amount of water to rinse with and spit out. Pursing and grimacing movements of the lips are also encouraged. An ideal impression material is one which is relatively fluid and can be easily extruded from beneath the registration blocks into the sulcus by moderate occlusal pressure. Zinc oxide/eugenol or light-bodied silicone are the materials of choice. When impressions are complete the blocks are sealed together in the retruded contact position by any convenient method (Fig. 2.6).

The technique is said to have the additional advantage that during the process of impression making any slight discrepancies in the jaw relations, resulting from points of premature contact of the rims, are eliminated. Occlusal irregularities might still be introduced at a later stage during the processing of the denture, and use of the technique will not compensate for lack of a final check record, either when the dentures are given to the patient or at review.

Although any differences in sulcus depth recorded by the open and closed-mouth techniques are not usually obvi-

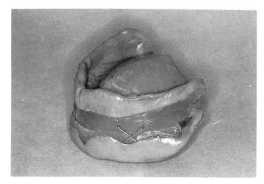

Fig. 2.6 Closed mouth impressions have been taken in registration blocks using a fluid silicone impression material.

ous to the operator there are other, sometimes readily observable, differences between the two types of impression.

One involves the changes produced by the coronoid processes which in the closed-mouth position lie laterally and distally to the maxillary tuberosity and form part of the lateral boundary of the coronomaxillary space, a region which has recently been described in detail.[9] When the mouth is opened the coronoid process is displaced forwards in relation to the maxilla as the condyles move downwards and forwards across the glenoid fossae. In this position, if the coronoid process is of the vertical type rather than flared laterally, it may fill the space buccal to the maxillary tuberosity and prevent impression material entering the sulcus (Fig. 2.7). When this complication is detected a special tray must be made and the periphery, which will be short in this region, extended into the sulcus using a functional trim material at the chairside. The final impression must then be made with the mouth sufficiently far closed to allow tray and impression material to enter the coronomaxillary space with ease.

Another change that follows opening of the mouth and forwards movement of the

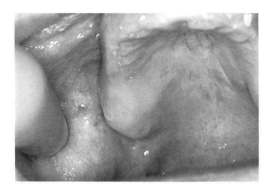

Fig. 2.7 The width of the maxillary sulcus posteriorly is limited by the presence of the coronoid process.

ramus of the mandible is a relative posterior displacement of the masseter muscle. Using the open-mouth technique the masseter does not influence the denture-bearing area. Using the closed-mouth technique, however, the periphery of a lower impression is often notched in the disto-buccal region,[10] the notching becoming more pronounced as occlusal pressure is exerted and the masseter, shortening further, exerts pressure on the periphery of the denture-bearing area through the buccinator. This is the reason for the common complaint at review of pain from the disto-buccal periphery of an apparently normally extended denture, the pain being made worse by increased biting pressure. Although most practitioners employ open mouth techniques with great success, knowledge of these two differences can permit them to anticipate at least two of the problems which occasionally occur and avoid any associated denture instability or patient discomfort.

Mucodisplacement and mucostatic techniques

The advantages and disadvantages of mucodisplacement and mucostatic techniques have been argued for some time. At first sight their rationales appear indisputable and the techniques free of complications. Hypothetically, a technique which involves compression and displacement of the denture-bearing tissues under a load comparable to that of occlusion allows a denture to be made which is more retentive during mastication, and a technique which records the tissues in an unloaded state allows a denture to be made which is more retentive during speech or when the tissues are unstrained. It follows that a denture made from a mucodisplacement impression fits best during mastication (when a devil's advocate might say the denture is being maintained in position not by the fluid film but principally by the applied muscle forces), and a denture made from a mucostatic impression fits best during speech (when some would say resistance to powerful displacing forces is not needed). The majority opinion at present favours the latter point of view and a recent review of prosthodontic standards advises that mucostatic techniques are used for the majority of normal cases.[11]

While the concept of uniform mucodisplacement of the tissues is simple to imagine it is difficult to achieve in practice. To record an impression of a denture-bearing area, the impression material must be capable of viscous flow as it is extruded under pressure from between the tray and the tissue surface. Hence, to record the tissues under pressure, materials of high viscosity are advised, such as dental composition, high viscosity silicones and stiff zinc oxide/eugenol. Like other fluids, impression materials will only flow under the influence of a pressure gradient from areas of high pressure to areas of low pressure or, in the case of an impression material, from the centre of the tray where pressure is highest to the periphery where pressure is least. Logically, so-called mucodisplacement techniques must give impressions which record the tissues as displaced by a gradient of pressure, most displacement occurring centrally and minimal displacement peripherally. An additional qualification is that unless the impression is removed from the mouth before any parts of it have set, then unless the entire mass of impression material sets simultaneously, the parts setting first will act as islands of high pressure and cause tissue distortion. For uniform mucodisplacement the tray must also maintain an equal spacing from the tissues to be recorded. If a local reduction of spacing takes place the forces required to cause flow through the narrowed ca-pillary-type space are greater and again greater local pressure is applied to the tis-sues. Finally, if the tray ever penetrates the impression material the underlying tissues will merely be forcibly conformed to the shape of the tray.

Rationally the only mucodisplacement impression material that can be recom-mended is one that flows continuously without setting, namely wax or other materials which soften at mouth temper-ature, and even materials of this type rec-ord tissues not under uniform pressure but under a pressure gradient. Correctly formulated impression waxes flow under pressure at mouth temperature and a range of waxes is produced for this pur-pose by manufacturers or can be made up by the interested practitioner.[12] By coating the fitting surface of an accu-rately close-fitting tray, and maintaining pressure on the tray in the mouth until flow around the entire periphery has been observed, it should be theoretically possible to record the denture-bearing tissues under pressure, with the qualifi-cation mentioned above that the rec-orded pressure, and hence tissue dis-placement, is greater centrally than peripherally. The use of impression com-position is subject to the same qualifi-cations, and to ensure that it acts in the required fashion it must be removed from the mouth while still warm enough to be capable of fluid flow.

Mucostatic impressions are easier to rationalize. To make an impression with-out displacement of the denture-bearing tissues, simply use a very fluid impression material and, while it sets, maintain the impression tray, under minimal pressure, without contact with the tissues. The types of impression material advised for this technique are plaster and the very fluid silicones. Skill is required to ensure that there is no contact between tray and tissues. To ensure that the tray does not penetrate the impression material it is advisable to use a slightly spaced (2–3 mm) tray. If stops are placed to permit precise location, the consequence is local areas of compression. When making the maxillary impression, to ensure patient comfort it is usually best to place a post dam on the fitting surface of the tray. It serves the double purpose of compress-ing the tissues in a region where com-pression is vital and inhibiting nausea by preventing extrusion of excess impression material into the pharynx.

Needless to say, there are few either truly mucodisplacing or mucostatic im-pression materials among the normal range employed in practice but despite this most complete dentures made with them have adequate retention, a finding reflecting credit on the average operator's skills and the average patient's tolerance.

Where fibrous replacement of the ridge has taken place—often seen in the max-illary anterior region—all except the most fluid of impression materials will cause flattening and displacement of the flabby tissues from their unstressed form. It may be argued that for best results the mobile fibrous tissues should be recorded under minimal pressure by means of a mucostatic technique, while the normal tissues elsewhere should be recorded with a more viscous material which can produce a moderate degree of functional mucodisplacement. This is most easily achieved in one stage using an impression material such as zinc oxide/eugenol or low viscosity silicone in a special tray which has been spaced and perforated only in the region of the fibrous tissue. The narrow capillary gap in unspaced areas, by restricting flow of the impression material, permits pressure to be applied, but the pressure will be relieved in the spaced areas.

A more sophisticated two-stage technique has been described for ensuring that pressure by the tray does not cause distortion of the mobile tissues.[13] On the model produced from the primary impression a close fitting acrylic special tray is made with a "window" over the mobile tissue. With the modified tray an impression is made in a suitable impression material, such as zinc oxide/eugenol, and any excess set material removed from the edges of the window. The impression is replaced in the mouth and a fluid impression material, either plaster or silicone, injected around the tissues exposed in the window (Fig. 2.8A, B and C). By maintaining pressure on the main part of the tray during the setting of the fluid impression material it is possible to produce a differential displacement impression.

A third method involves splinting the mobile tissues while the main impression is made. After making a preliminary impression in a fluid material, such as alginate, a model is cast of the relatively undistorted ridge. Over the model is made a spaced (3–4 mm) rigid tray and an impression of the model taken, in the tray, using composition. As a preliminary step, before taking the final impression

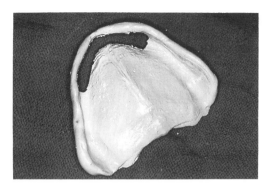

Fig. 2.8A An impression has been made with zinc oxide/eugenol in a windowed, close fitting special tray.

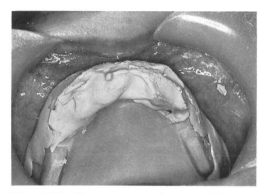

Fig. 2.8B The tray is replaced and the impression completed in impression plaster.

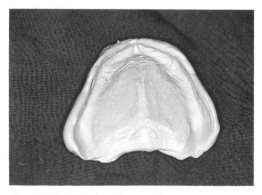

Fig. 2.8C The final impression.

the periphery of the composition is carefully softened and functionally trimmed. For the final impression the composition over the hard areas is softened with a flame before the tray is seated under heavy pressure. By preforming the impression material in this way the original undistorted shape of the mobile tissues is retained while the tissues more capable of denture support are recorded in a displaced state.

Selective (peripheral) pressure techniques

From the mechanics of denture retention it appears that the impression most likely to ensure maximum retention is one which causes slight compression of the tissues at the periphery, so reducing the distance between the future denture and its supporting tissues (see equation 1) and increasing the force required to shear the saliva film. This is said to be confirmed by the great increase in retention achieved when a post dam is added to the palate of an otherwise non-retentive maxillary denture.[14] Nevertheless, care has to be taken that the pressure exerted at the periphery does not exceed tissue tolerance or impede muscle action. Much of the periphery of a denture is situated adjacent to muscle insertions and overextension will cause instability, or if retention is especially good, pain.

Two types of material have been specially developed to ensure slight peripheral overextension and compression. The first of these functional trim materials is a slow-setting poly butylmethacrylate resin (a moderately stiff mix of Total Hard works well). The technique for use varies in detail whether a maxillary or mandibular impession is being made. For the maxillary impression a close fitting special tray is reduced by 2–3 mm from its correct functional extension into

the sulcus as determined by inspection. The functional trim material is mixed and applied with a spatula as a beading to the outside of the tray periphery. After inserting the tray the setting material can be made to flow into the sulcus by external digital pressure via the cheeks and lips. the material must be viscous enough to distend the sulcus slightly while setting and once the material has set—a process accelerated by removing the impression and immersing it in hot water—the impression is completed with a wash of zinc oxide/eugenol or silicone.

The mandibular impression is recorded by first applying functional trim to the entire fitting surface of a close fitting, reduced, special tray. On insertion, pressure is exerted on the tray to force the functional trim to the edge of the tray where it fills the sulcus. Vigorous muscle trimming will produce a functionally extended periphery and the impression is perfected by a wash in a fluid material.

Recently a silicone putty has been developed specifically as a functional trim material (Xantopren Function, Bayer, W. Germany). It can be used for mandibular and maxillary impressions when it is used in exactly the same way as the poly (butyl methacrylate) type but like all silicones needs to be bonded to the tray with a special adhesive. The setting time is prolonged (8–10 minutes) to allow adaptation to the functional shape of the sulcus. A perfecting wash is taken (Fig. 2.9A and B) if necessary in another specially developed silicone (Xantopren Mucosa).

The classical way of making a mandibular impression with peripheral compression is that advocated by Fournet and Tuller in 1937.[15] After making an accurate, close-fitting special tray the edges are reduced until they are 2–3 mm short of the functional depth of the sulcus. The periphery is then extended to

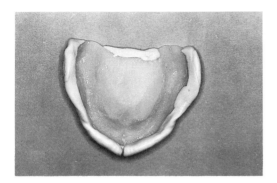

Fig. 2.9A A close fitting special tray extended with silicone putty into the functional sulcus.

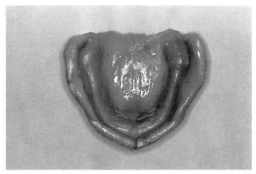

Fig. 2.9B The impression is completed with a wash of fluid silicone.

the full functional depth by addition of softened Greenstick or similar thermoplastic material (Fig. 2.10). Care is taken to ensure that the amount of peripheral compression is uniform by repeated warming, reinsertion and functional trimming of the added material. A maxillary tray is treated in the same way and a functional post dam added in the region of the junction of hard and soft palate, before a wash is taken to complete the impressions. Pain from the denture-bearing surface adjacent to the periphery, especially in the mylohyoid ridge region, can sometimes follow insertion of a denture made from this type of impression. To prevent this, and ensure that any extra pressure is directed peripherally and not over the bone adjacent to the periphery at the site of the thermoplastic addition, allow unimpeded flow of the impression material towards the periphery by thinning the internal aspects of the extension with a sharp knife.

Thermoplastic materials are difficult to maintain at a uniform viscosity and cool areas can cause sites of excess pressure where the overlying wash impression material will be penetrated. A simple means of producing an impression with slight peripheral compression which over-

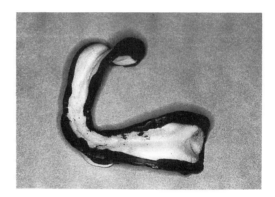

Fig. 2.10 A close fitting special tray functionally extended with Greenstick composition.

comes this difficulty is that advocated by Hobkirk[16] as a routine impression method. Again, close fitting special trays are made and reduced to a point just short of the visible sulcus. After extending the entire periphery apart from the post dam region with Greenstick composition, an initial impression is taken, applying a mix of zinc oxide/eugenol to the edge of the tray. The action of inserting the tray then drives the impression material into the sulcus where it is trimmed by functional movements. The impression is completed with a wash of zinc oxide/eugenol after reducing with a scalpel any areas where the underlying composition is seen to penetrate (Fig. 2.11A and B).

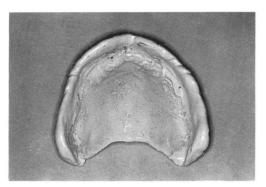

Fig. 2.11A After making a functional addition to the periphery in Greenstick composition a preliminary impression of the periphery is made in zinc oxide/eugenol.

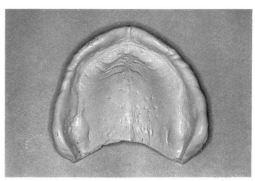

Fig. 2.11B After reducing any areas where perforation has occurred the impression is completed with a wash of zinc oxide/eugenol.

A modified form of selective compression has been advised for the maxillary molar region. Sometimes considerable alveolar resorption has taken place here, and to augment retention a facial seal can be created laterally between the mucosa of the cheek and the buccal surface of the denture periphery. The technique seeks to avoid the error of extending the periphery too far vertically and so displacing the insertion of the buccinator muscle and involves first building out the tray laterally in the molar region with a material such as composition or Peripheral Seal, before an overall wash impression is taken. If the patient can tolerate the thickened periphery the contact established buccally between the polished surface and the cheek mucosa is said to provide extra security for the border seal. When using this method care must be taken at the impression stage that the extension to the tray does not impede movement of the coronoid process of the mandible.

Techniques to improve stability

For complete dentures, stability may be defined in terms of their ability to resist functional forces displacing them away from the denture-bearing surface other than at right angles to it. The prerequisite for maximizing denture stability would appear to ensure that the artificial teeth are set in their functional position, namely the site once occupied by the natural teeth. It is hypothesized that here they occupy the neutral zone where the forces exerted outwards on the teeth by the tongue are balanced by forces exerted inwards by the lips and cheeks. This is not to imply that the opposing forces are always balanced. The neutral zone only exists as a mean position and even over short periods of time the site of the neutral zone will change as muscle movements cause local changes in the point of balance. While techniques designed to define the neutral zone for the purposes of tooth location may help provide increased stability, any denture must have enough intrinsic retention to resist the momentary displacing forces caused by imbalanced muscle action.

Most clinical techniques for improving stability in this way are derived from the anthropoidal pouch technique described by Fish.[17] The original method established not only the site of the teeth but the shape of the functional denture space which was duplicated to provide a model for the shape of the polished surfaces of the future denture. To simplify the procedures it is used only for the mandibular denture. The first stage is to make an acceptably retentive maxillary denture (a correctly made maxillary denture possesses enough retention to resist most destabilizing muscle forces). Subsequently, the mandibular functional denture space is recorded as determined by the interaction between the oral musculature and the retentive maxillary denture.

After taking impressions of the mandibular denture-bearing area and the occlusal surface of the maxillary denture, a preliminary registration is made of the jaw relations to ensure that the denture space is recorded at the correct face height. A special tray is constructed which not only covers the denture-bearing area but projects vertically to maintain contact with the occlusal surface of the maxillary denture at the correct face height. The projection also serves to retain the impression material and may consist of wire loops or acrylic supports. If acrylic is chosen it should give support only in the premolar region, otherwise the free movement of impression material will be hindered. When the tray has been corrected, all its surfaces are coated with alginate, it is seated and the patient who has been trained in the actions required, is asked to perform functional movements such as smiling, pouting and tongue projecting, before coming to rest in the retruded contact position.

The impression is removed, a model cast to the fitting surface and after placing a model of the maxillary denture into position, sectional casts are made to the buccal, labial and lingual surfaces. A try-in is made by removing the impression, laying down a shellac base on the model and filling the denture space with liquid

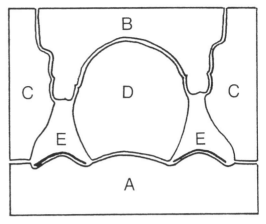

Fig. 2.12 Cross-section of sectional casts made to a neutral zone impression which has been removed. A, mandibular model, B, model of maxillary denture, C and D, buccal and lingual casts, E, shellac base.

wax (Fig. 2.12). After dismantling the casts the wax teeth are replaced by appropriate denture teeth articulated to the upper model. If the try-in is satisfactory the denture is processed in the normal way.

Variations on the basic technique have been described. The commonest is to use the prepared tray to first make an impression of the denture-bearing surface only. With the tray *in situ* and while the patient is asked to maintain the retruded contact position, impression material is injected via a syringe into the denture space. Alginate, plaster and silicone are the materials of choice and permit extensive records of the buccal and lingual soft tissues. Alternatively, a completely conventional denture technique can be used, with the exception that the mandibular registration block is made from impression wax.[18] After establishing the correct face height the wax rim remains in place for 5–10 minutes to adapt to the neutral zone while the patient performs functional movements at intervals. Care has to be taken that the face height is not reduced during this time. While the latter technique may well record the correct neutral zone for the teeth, the adaptation of the lingual and buccal surfaces of the future base to the denture space is less well marked. In addition, the large amount of wax required is a considerable expense if a proprietary brand of impression wax is chosen.

A more recent analysis of neutral zone procedures casts doubt on their usefulness for all cases.[19] While the study established the value of biometric guides in determining tooth positions, it also re-affirmed some much earlier work[20] which claimed that the experimentally determined neutral zone lay further buccally than the natural teeth and that in life, to aid swallowing, the tongue had to be constrained by the dental arch. The conclusion was that artificial teeth set in a neutral zone determined by unrestrained muscle function would lie too far buccally for optimum functional efficiency. It was nevertheless allowed that neutral zone techniques may be helpful when treating skeletal relationships other than class I, especially for siting the mandibular teeth. Unfortunately the only clinical trial to date which attempted to relate post-insertion patient comfort with whether or not a neutral zone technique was used, gave ambiguous results.[21] Not only were the subjects selected from a dissatisfied group (so eliminating all patients who had been satisfied by conventional techniques), but the impression technique more resembled a record of the functional periphery.

Other impression techniques for improving stability involve extending the lingual periphery of the mandibular denture into the retromylohyoid and sublingual spaces. The retromylohyoid space is a cleft of variable size sandwiched between the distal attachment of the mylohyoid muscle to the mylohyoid line,

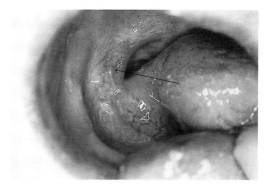

Fig. 2.13 Posterior boundary of the mandibular lingual sulcus with the tongue retracted medially. An arrow indicates the palatoglossal arch.

and the body of the tongue in the third molar region. Its lateral wall is the mucous membrane overlying the mylohyoid muscle, and its floor the mucous membrane reflection as it turns from the mylohyoid muscle to cover the muscles of the tongue and forms the medial wall. With the tongue protruded, its posterior boundary is the mucous membrane covering the palatoglossal arch (Fig. 2.13) with, near the floor, a slip of the superior constrictor running medially from its attachment to the mandible below the inferior end of the pterygo-mandibular raphe to its insertion into the muscles of the tongue.

Any extension into this space must be made with the tongue protruded so that the mylohyoid, palatoglossus and superior constrictor muscles are actively forming the borders. At rest, impression material can displace the lax mylohyoid and by running beneath the mylohyoid ridge, occupy an undercut which causes pain if reproduced in the denture. With the tongue protruded the mylohyoid space is very much reduced in extent but small extensions into the cleft can be made provided that the final impression is supported by a rigid functionally developed extension to the tray. The

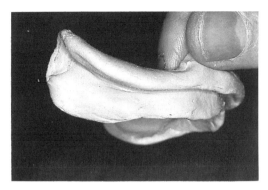

Fig. 2.14 Extension of a mandibular impression into the retromylohyoid space.

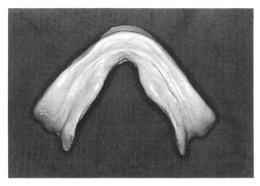

Fig. 2.15 Mandibular impression showing sublingual extensions.

extension to the denture, which is directed medially and inferiorly, acts as a stabilizer by supporting the base of the tongue (Fig. 2.14).

A sublingual extension[22] is made horizontally in the premolar and incisor region, filling the potential space between the floor of the mouth and the ventral surface of the tongue. Like the retromylohyoid extension, the sublingual extension is recorded with the tongue protruded in an active position and serves to stabilize the tongue by providing an anterior rest (Fig. 2.15).

Extensions into both spaces are best made by addition of functional trimming material (Greenstick composition is suitable) to the special tray while the tongue is protruded to touch the corner of the mouth at the side opposite to the extension. The working impression is made after satisfactory extensions have been formed. Both sides can be recorded simultaneously by protruding the tongue or making side-to-side functional movements.

Removal of impressions from the mouth

Impression materials such as the reversible and irreversible hydrocolloids and the elastomers are visco-elastic and their recovery from a strain is time dependent. Certain precautions have to be taken if an undercut is to be recorded accurately. The impression must be removed from the mouth as rapidly as possible so that the strain rate is high and the amount of permanent residual strain minimal. Before casting a model the impression should be allowed to stand while any further elastic recovery takes place. Ideally this period should be as long as possible, but 10–15 minutes is a sensible time.

References

1. Halperin, A.R., Graser, G.N., Rogoff, G.S. and Plekavitch, E.J. *Mastering the Art of Complete Dentures.* Chicago: Quintessence Publishing Co. Ltd., 1988.
2. Linstrom, R.E., Pawelchak, J., Heyd, A. and Tarbet, W.J. Physical-chemical aspects of denture retention and stability— a review of the literature. *J Prosthet Dent* **42**:371–375, 1979.
3. Barbenel, J.C. Physical retention of full dentures. *J Prosthet Dent* **26**:592–600, 1971.
4. Ellis, B., Lamb, D.J. and Al Nakash, S. The composition and rheology of denture adhesives. *J Dent* **8**:109–118, 1980.

5. Defay, R., Prigogine, I., Bellemans, A. and Everett, D.H. Surface Tension and Absorption, London: Longmans, p. 7, 1966.

6. O'Brien, W.J. and Ryge, G. Wettability of poly(methyl methacrylate) treated with carbon tetrachloride. *J Prosthet Dent* **15**:304–308, 1965.

7. Boucher, L.J., Ellinger, C., Lutes, M. and Hickey, J.C. The effects of a microlayer of silica on the retention of mandibular complete dentures. *J Prosthet Dent* **10**:516–624, 1960.

8. Hargreaves, A.S. and Foster, M.A. Hydrocryl: an aid to retention. *J Dent* **4**:33–61, 1976.

9. Arbree, N.S., Yurkstas, A.A. and Kronman, J.H. The coronomaxillary space: Literature review and anatomic description. *J Prosthet Dent* **53**:186–190, 1987.

10. Pendleton, E.C. The anatomy of the maxillae from the point of view of a full denture prosthesis. *J Am Dent Assoc* **19**:543–572, 1932.

11. Academy of Denture Prosthetics, Principles, concepts and practices in prosthodontics. *J Prosthet Dent* **61**:88–109, 1989.

12. McCrorie, J. Impression waxes. *Br Dent J* **152**:95–96, 1982.

13. Osborne, J. Two impression techniques for mobile fibrous ridge. *Br Dent J* 117:392–394, 1964.

14. Moghadam, B.K. and Scandrett, F.R. A technique for adding the posterior palatal seal. *J Prosthet Dent* **32**:443–447, 1974.

15. Fournet, S.C. and Tuller, C.S. A revolutionary mechnical principle utilised to produce full lower dentures surpassing in stability the best modern upper dentures. *J Am Dent Assoc* **11**:16–20, 1937.

16. Hobkirk, J.A. *Complete Dentures*. Bristol: Wright, p. 44, 1986.

17. Fish, W. *Principles of Full Denture Prosthesis*. 6th Ed. London: Staples Press, 1964.

18. Murphy, W.M. The neutral zone and the polished surface of full dentures. *Dent Pract* **16**:244–248, 1966.

19. Neill, D.J. and Glaysher, J.K.L. Identifying the denture space. *J Oral Rehabil* **9**:259–277, 1982.

20. Dixon, D.A. An investigation into the influence of soft tissues on tooth position. *Br Soc Study Ortho Tr* **10**:89–92, 1959.

21. Barrenas, L. and Odman, P. Myodynamic and conventional construction of complete dentures: a comprehensive study of comfort and function. *J Oral Rehabil* **16**:457–465, 1989.

22. Fish, E.W. Tongue space in full denture construction. *Br Dent J* **83**:137–142, 1947.

Chapter 3

Technical Support

Impressions should be cast soon after they are made, but a delay period of about 15 minutes is desirable to allow any visco-elastic rebound to take place. In a busy surgery the time can be employed in carrying out decontamination procedures. When it is anticipated that distortion of an impression might take place, either during transport to the technician or while waiting for it to be collected, the impression should be cast immediately and a small amount of die stone kept in a side room for just this purpose. Technical instructions have to be detailed and specific and cover the requirements for casting models, the type of special trays and amount of spacing, and the materials and form of the registration blocks.

Disinfection and sterilization procedures

We live in a health conscious age and the expectations of our patients to be treated under safe conditions must be satisfied. It is now difficult to justify not having an autoclave to sterilize reusable materials. The current spectres are AIDS and hepatitis B, and these two conditions must at least be thanked for stimulating concern for cross-infection control! Although the virus responsible for AIDS is relatively

easily destroyed by normal precautions, the hepatitis B virus is more difficult to kill and it is important that all dental personnel, either directly or indirectly concerned with patient treatment, take the prophylactic measure of being immunized against this organism.

Apart from the normal requirements for control of cross-infection in the surgery, the practice of prosthodontics involves a third person who must be protected, the dental technician. The most obvious way for this to be done is by preventing infected material leaving the surgery environment, which at this stage involves disinfecting or sterilizing all impressions and their associated trays. Fortunately, the American Dental Association has produced useful guidelines to how this can be achieved.[1]

Of the two, disinfection is faster and involves eliminating all viable bacteria (including tubercle bacilli) and deactivating any viruses (including hepatitis B). Usually 0.5% or 1% hypochlorite, or 2% glutaraldehyde, is used although there are reports that glutaraldehyde causes skin sensitivity and its use is governed by the Control of Substances Hazardous to Health (COSSH) regulations. Disinfection results after immersion for 15 minutes. Early work[2] showed the surface of the impression materials to be relatively unaffected by a period of immersion as brief as this, although a later study[3] showed that some types of alginate are susceptible to damage. Susceptibility to damage by disinfectant solutions appears to vary between makes, and it is sensible to choose a brand without this disadvantage. Although specific tests have not been carried out, it is also to be expected that the reversible and irreversible hydrocolloids will undergo slight dimensional changes following immersion in an aqueous medium for the lengths of time needed for disinfection.

Prior to immersion all impressions and their trays must be rinsed in running water to remove traces of blood or mucus, otherwise the action of the disinfecting agent is adversely affected and effective immersion times cannot be guaranteed. After immersion the impression is again rinsed in running water before being placed in a polythene bag and taken to the technician.

Immersion procedures have disadvantages. Glutaraldehyde is expensive and hypochlorite has a smell which some find offensive. A suggested means of disinfection which overcomes these disadvantages is a "hard surface" chlorhexidine/isopropyl alcohol antiseptic spray, which is normally used on working surfaces and is applied to impressions after they have been rinsed clean of debris and contaminants.[4] The method is effective and can be applied not only to impressions but to all work going to and coming from the laboratory.

Sterilization is more difficult and involves eliminating all living organisms including spores. Immersion for 10–15 hours in a chemical disinfectant is necessary, and under these conditions the surfaces of many impression materials are severely affected, including the alginates, the polysulphides, polyethers, dental composition and zinc oxide/eugenol. If sterilization must be ensured, as in the case of

a known hepatitis carrier, the only satisfactory impression materials would appear to be the silicone elastomers, which have long been known to withstand sterilization routines of this nature.[5] A further problem encountered with sterilization in hypochlorite solutions for such prolonged time is that metal trays undergo accelerated corrosion.

Because disinfection and sterilization of impressions are inconvenient, a number of alternatives have been investigated. The first was an alginate containing a disinfectant. Although an excellent idea in theory, the antiseptic (didecyl dimethyl ammonium chloride) was found to be relatively ineffective against viruses such as polio virus and herpes simplex.[6] Further, alginate is transported to the mouth in a tray and even if the alginate were rendered safe it would still be necessary to disinfect the tray with some form of hard-surface antiseptic spray. More recently, disinfecting die stones have been introduced.[7] While their physical properties are comparable with normal die stones, and their disinfecting properties appear adequate, the person handling or casting an infected impression would still appear to be at risk. Although using a disinfecting die stone would avoid the need to disinfect the models at subsequent stages, it would not overcome the initial problem of contamination which would be solved only if the DSA and technician could be persuaded to wear gloves when handling and casting impressions.

The measures mentioned above apply equally to all other work going to the laboratory and to work coming from the laboratory to the surgery. Work from a laboratory should be at least disinfected and where the patient may be immunocompromised, sterilization of all work is mandatory. Fortunately the majority of materials used in prosthetic technology are resistant to damage by the disinfecting regimes mentioned above.

Transport of impressions

Set impression materials vary in their capacity to undergo strain without permanent distortion. If impressions are to be stored or transported, the conditions for storage or transport have to be such as to prevent any change in shape.

Zinc oxide/eugenol withstands stresses well, especially if the impression is supported beneath its entire periphery by a close-fitting rigid tray. For the purposes of transport, only an impact resistant container is needed. Silicone elastomers are visco-elastic and distort permanently if prolonged stresses are applied and silicone impressions must be well protected during storage and transport. While addition-cured silicones may be stored for prolonged periods without undergoing permanent dimensional change, the condensation-cured type are less stable and must not only be well supported in storage but should not be allowed to remain for more than 24 hours without being cast.

The hydrocolloids, whether reversible or irreversible, are least resistant to applied stresses or prolonged storage. Not only must they be well supported and protected but the outer layer of wrapping has to be impervious to water. If gain or loss of water occurs, dimensional changes follow. Because they are so susceptible to dimensional change, it is these types of impression for which immediate casting is so important, and a DSA should be trained for the task of casting an impression, if necessary leaving its basing to be done by the technician at a more convenient time.

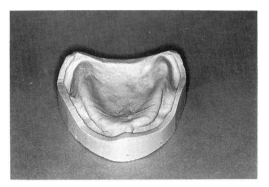

Fig. 3.1 A maxillary model showing adequate reproduction of the sulcus.

Technical instructions

Models

Because primary and working impressions serve different purposes there are slight differences in the appearance of the types of model cast from them. The model produced from a primary impression should allow access for the technician to the entire periphery so that an accurately extended special tray can be made. The part of the model which extends beyond the impression surface —the "land"—should be reduced to an appropriate level. A working impression, on the other hand, records not only the denture-bearing area but also the reflection of the sulcus so that the border seal can be augmented by close contact of the future polished surface with the soft tissues. The working model should be cast in such a way as to record the sulcus and be carried round the full extent of the border onto the future polished surface (Fig. 3.1). Beading of the impression with soft wax prior to casting helps define the surfaces to be recorded. Boxing-in the impression with sheet wax is an additional aid which restrains the plaster and cuts down on technical work. Although the production of a fully extended registration block and try-in is made more difficult by partial enclosure of the sulcus in this way, the need for accurate reproduction of the periphery takes precedence.

Special trays

To ensure an accurate record of the denture-bearing surface and a functional record of the periphery it is usual to take a second set of impressions in special, custom made trays, either spaced or unspaced. These are designed on the primary model and are adjusted in the mouth, as necessary, to ensure an accurate fit. When no undercuts have to be recorded, the trays can be a close, unspaced fit on the model and no restrictions need to be placed on the choice of impression material. If the surfaces to be recorded are undercut, elastic impression materials have to be used and the degree of spacing of the tray must be influenced by the properties of the proposed material.

When elastic impression materials are disengaged from an undercut that part of the impression material which enters the undercut is distorted in a mixture of shear and compression. Whether or not the impression material recovers its original dimensions (i.e. does not undergo permanent strain) depends on the rate at which the impression material is strained (i.e. the rate at which it is removed from the undercut) and the more rapid the rate the less the chance of permanent distortion. At the same time the shear stress must not be great enough to exceed the tear strength of the impression material. With any selected impression material the strains will be greater with deeper undercuts and greater spacing is needed to reduce the chances of tearing. Tear strengths of silicones are greater than

those of alginate and hence less spacing is required.

The presence and depth of undercuts vary in different sites of the same patient's residual ridge. It would be tedious to provide a tray with a mixture of spaced and unspaced parts and so it is customary to design trays with an overall spacing equal to the maximum amount required. When using alginate for undercuts in the anterior and premolar region this can usually be provided by blocking out undercuts with wax then providing a spacing of 3–4 mm. This takes into account that usually part of any undercut is bone and part mucoperiosteum, and mucoperiosteum will itself distort to allow removal of impressions. Following the above rule gives good results in most cases. At times, however, very large undercuts occur in the maxillary tuberosity region and surgical reduction cannot be performed because it is contraindicated by the patient's health or inclination. Extra spacing will then be needed in this region but may be limited by the extent to which interference with the coronoid processes occurs. The greater tear strength of silicone permits less extra spacing.

Two more problems may arise when removing impressions from undercut areas, the first resulting from the effects of the shear component applied to the impression material when it is displaced from the undercut. When withdrawing impressions from large undercuts shear forces are applied to the impression which may be sufficient to detach the impression material from its tray. For this reason it is wise when dealing with spaced trays to adopt a "belt and braces" approach and ensure that not only are retention holes cut in the tray, but a tray adhesive is used.

The other problem is one which can occur when large undercuts are recorded using an impression material which while sufficiently elastic, has a high modulus of elasticity when set. Under these circumstances the force required to remove the tray, while not great enough to permanently strain the impression, may be beyond the tolerance or pain threshold of the patient. This is most likely to occur when recording bony undercuts with an addition-cured silicone. For our patients' sakes it is probably best to ensure that when using silicones to record undercuts in complete denture prosthodontics, only the condensation-cured type are employed despite their lesser degree of long-term stability.

A special form of tray, a biometric tray, can be designed to take into account the resorption that follows tooth loss and, hypothetically, record the sulcus in its pre-extraction site.[8] Models are first cast from impressions made in oversize stock trays, the flanges of which give the degree of support to the surrounding musculature which resorption has deprived it of. The design of the upper tray is complex and depends on identifying on the model the biometric marker of the lingual gingival margin. The tray is constructed with the periphery spaced 6, 8, 10, and 12 mm buccal to the lingual gingival margin in the incisor, canine, premolar and molar regions, respectively. Because it is thought that a preliminary impression might deepen the sulcus excessively, and that the sulcus will be shallower when supported by the biometric tray, the tray is extended into the sulcus no further than 5 mm beyond the muco-gingival line. Over the palate the tray remains unspaced.

Biometric lower trays are similarly designed to support the soft tissues, but do so by a vertical extension of the body of the tray. In the incisor region this slopes forward slightly to support the lower lip and in the molar region it bulges buccally to support the buccinator.

All special trays are provided with handles for their control. Generally the handles are near vertical at the base where they might contact the lips but may be of any convenient shape once there is no longer a risk of interference. Vertical finger supports in the mandibular premolar region allow a tray to be maintained in position without the finger tips distorting the sulcus.

Record blocks

A record block comprises a base and a rim. The base is normally made of a thermoplastic material which can be easily formed by heat to the surface of the working model. Shellac is a popular choice and having a softening temperature well above 37°C does not significantly change shape in the mouth. Wax can be used for ease and cheapness, but its low softening temperature means that the operator must work quickly—perhaps too quickly for a high standard of work. Autopolymerizing acrylic resin is another alternative, but without great care the polymerization shrinkage which takes place produces an inaccurate fit.

The accuracy of the registration process depends to a considerable extent on the accurate fitting of the base of the record block. While well formed ridges give a degree of stability which promotes accurate jaw relations, when alveolar resorption is marked an accurate registration depends entirely on the intrinsic retention of the base. It is pointless attempting to record jaw relations when retention of the base is poor. If optimum results are to be achieved and extreme alveolar resorption has taken place, permanent acrylic bases are made on the working models. They are then used as the base for the rim and later the try-in. To avoid subsequent distortion of the bases during the processing stage the

71

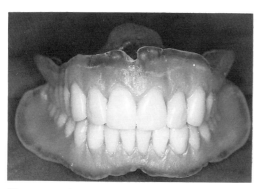

Fig. 3.2 Complete dentures processed on clear acrylic resin permanent bases.

remainder of the denture is processed by a prolonged cure at 70°C (Fig. 3.2).

It is possible to use autopolymerizing acrylic resin instead of heat-cured but porosity can follow. After insertion of such a denture, the high level of residual monomer can be troublesome in sensitive patients, and in the long term discolouration of the pigments may occur.

Wax is the usual material used for rims. Although it softens at mouth temperature the bulk of the rim resists distortion and cooling the block at intervals helps maintain stability. At times thermoplastic materials such as composition have been advised, but the difficulties encountered in modification of a rim of this material outweigh the extra stability. To help speed the registration process the maxillary and mandibular rims can be made 22 mm and 18 mm high, respectively, from the deepest part of the anterior sulcus to the edge of the rim. These measurements correspond to the mean dimensions found in life.

References

1. Council on Dental Materials, Instruments and Equipment. Infection control recommendations for the dental office and the dental laboratory. *J Am Dent Assoc* **116**:241–248, 1988.
2. Herrera, S.P. and Merchent, V.A. Dimensional stability of dental impressions after immersion disinfection. *J Am Dent Assoc* **113**:419–422, 1986.
3. Tullner, J.B., Commette, J.A. and Moon, P.C. Linear dimensional changes in dental impressions after immersion in disinfectant solutions. *J Prosthet Dent* **60**:725–728, 1988.
4. Welfare, R.D. and Wright, S.M. Fundamentals of prosthetic practice. *Br Dent J* **167**:282–285, 1989.
5. Storer, R. and McCabe, J.F. An investigation of methods available for sterilising impressions. *Br Dent J* **151**:217–219, 1981.
6. Tyler, R., Tobias, R.S., Ayliffe, G.A.T. and Browne, R.M. An in vitro study of the antiviral properties of an alginate impression material impregnated with disinfectant. *J Dent* **17**:137–139, 1989.
7. Donovan, T. and Chee, W.W.L Preliminary investigation of a disinfected gypsum die stone. *Int J Prosthet* **2**:245–248, 1989.
8. Watt, D.M. and MacGregor, A.R. *Designing Complete Dentures*. 2nd Ed. Bristol: Wright, pp 160–165, 1986.

Chapter 4

Registration

While each step in the registration process has unique problems the overall problem is one of communication with the patient and the technician. Normally communication is by word, either written or spoken, supplemented by diagram or picture. Such forms suffice for communications with the patient, but during the course of registering the jaw relations the concepts to be transmitted to the technician are so complex that they are inadequate and a specially modified construction—the registration block—has to be employed. By modifying the wax rims the operator prescribes precise instructions which determine the support for the soft tissues, the static and dynamic jaw relations and the site of the teeth. Written instructions and possibly diagrams can supplement the information and prescribe the arrangement, colour, size and shape of the teeth. So long as there are problems associated with clinical procedures, their magnitude can only be made worse by poor communication. All too frequently we assume the technician to have information which can only be acquired by clinical access to the patient. In addition to providing precise instructions, if facilities are available, and especially if instructions are complex, we should not hesitate to involve the technician at the chairside. The consequent

improvements in information transfer and personal interest are substantial.

Soft tissue support

The first part of the registration process is to adjust the wax rims to provide the degree of soft tissue support required. Conventionally a hot metal plate is used for melting away surplus wax. The metal plate can be heated in a gas flame but in these safety-conscious days, clinicians are aware of the dangers of working with latex gloves in the vicinity of a naked flame and the use of a hot-air jet is becoming more popular.[1]

Upper lip

The correct degree of support for the upper lip can be difficult to determine and patients sometimes ask for abnormal amounts of support to be provided in order to "improve" their appearance and eliminate signs of ageing. To preserve the illusion of reality, support can only be given in those sites where loss of tissue has taken place. It is wrong, therefore, to support the upper lip by thickening the labial surface of the registration block generally and imagine that when this has been reproduced in the denture a normal

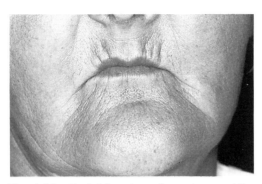

Fig. 4.1A Radial lines have formed around the mouth.

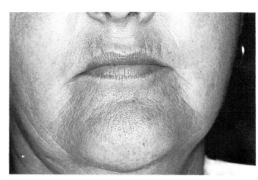

Fig. 4.1B A complete denture has been provided with adequate lip support, but the remnants of the radial lines are still visible.

appearance will result. The tissues to be replaced are tooth and alveolar bone. The proportion of alveolar bone decreases towards the tooth apex and hence at the reflection of the mucosa in the deepest part of the sulcus little bone has been lost and minimal tissue replacement is required. Thickening this region will give the appearance of inflammatory swelling rather than natural support.

Correctly situated lip support can improve those signs of ageing made worse by tooth loss but some signs cannot be rectified, and if radial lines have formed around the mouth no tolerable degree of lip support can eliminate them completely (Fig. 4.1A and B). To some extent the visibility of deep naso-labial folds can be reduced by increasing lip support but best results are achieved not by increasing support in the canine region but by increasing it in the central incisor region. This will have the effect of drawing the upper lip forwards, reducing the apparent depth of the naso-labial folds and ensuring that no unsightly excess support is given over the canine eminence.

To help ensure that the degree of upper lip support is correct a number of guidelines have been suggested. It has been proposed that with correct support of the upper lip the angle between the philtrum and the columella of the nose should be approximately 90°. This holds good for many patients but is inappropriate for those with a prominent columella—a situation common in class II cases—when the angle should be greater than 90°. As a corollary, the angle between the philtrum and the columella should be less than 90° when there is a class III jaw relationship and a relative maxillary retrusion (Fig. 4.2). The clinician should be prepared therefore, to use the rule in "average" cases but modify it in accordance with his judgement.

It has been suggested that if lip support is correct then, when viewed from the front, the oral mucosa of the lip should be just visible when the lips are slightly apart. Again, while the rule is helpful with "average" patients its value is lost when treating unusual cases, e.g. skeletal class III cases or patients with prominent lips.

The palatine (incisive) papilla is a useful landmark for judging the likely site of the upper anterior teeth and the correct degree of lip support. Extensive studies[2] have shown that when the natural teeth are not unduly proclined or retroclined, the centre of the palatine papilla lies 8–10

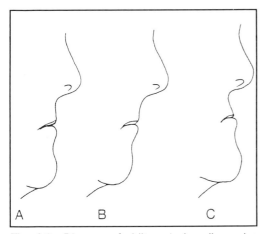

Fig. 4.2 Diagram of philtrum/columella angles for three cases: A, class I, B, class II, C, class III.

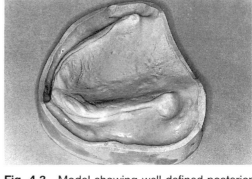

Fig. 4.3 Model showing well defined posterior lingual gingival margin remnants.

mm behind the labial surfaces of the maxillary central incisors, and its distal margin is intersected by a line passing through the centres of the canines. Following loss of the teeth and the associated alveolar resorption, slight relative changes occur and the palatine papilla is displaced forwards its distal margin now occupying that site where once the centre was. The palatine papilla is easily visible on the fitting surface of a well adapted registration block and by adjusting a pair of dividers to the required distance the amount of lip support can be quickly checked.

While landmarks are available which permit correct positioning of the maxillary anterior teeth the posterior teeth are more of a problem. In some patients the remnants of the lingual marginal gingivae of the posterior teeth remain visible on the model as a depressed line (Fig. 4.3). Due to the resorption and flattening that follows tooth loss the line lies 2–3 mm buccal to the position occupied in life. When this landmark is available it can be made use of and the wax rim trimmed back until, in the sagittal plane, its buccal surface lies 8, 10, or 12 mm further buccal to the gingival remnant in the canine,

premolar and molar regions, respectively.

A recent development[3] in research into biometric markers has identified an interesting correlation. The width of the tips of the lateral arms of a gothic arch or arrow-head tracing in dentate subjects has been shown to be proportional to the distance between the buccal cusps of pairs of contralateral maxillary posterior teeth. Thus the gothic arch width has been shown to be in the ratio 1:2 with that of the intercanine width, with smaller ratios for more posterior teeth. Such a relationship is not as unlikely as it appears. It is probable that lateral rotation of the mandible, as recorded by the trace, is limited by contact of the coronoid processes with the zygomatic process of the maxilla and the trace is a record of the maxillary width. The use of this finding will be considerably enhanced if it is found to be equally valid in edentulous subjects after resorption has taken place.

Lower lip

Although biometric markers exist to aid the clinician site maxillary teeth in the position they occupied in life, the problem of siting mandibular teeth is less easily overcome. It is tempting to trim the wax record block so that the future anterior teeth will lie over the ridge and secure maximum mechanical stability, although at the expense of poor appearance. Most experienced clinicians teach that for optimum functional stability the mandibular anterior teeth must be in the place they occupied in life and as most resorption in the mandibular anterior region takes place labially a position 2–3 mm anterior to the crest of the residual alveolar ridge is recommended, and the wax record block should be trimmed accordingly. Where resorption has taken place to such an extent that it is difficult to be certain where the crest of the residual ridge is, it is best to rely on direct inspection of the lips in profile. Assuming that the maxillary rim has been correctly trimmed, then undue prominence of the lower lip caused by the block being insufficiently trimmed is easily indentified; overtrimming of the block is more difficult to be certain about but usually results in a slight relative prominence of the upper lip.

Tooth visibility

Most textbooks advise that the labial incisal edge of the maxillary wax rim and consequently the incisal edges of the maxillary incisor teeth should be level with the lower border of the upper lip. Adhering to this rule will give good results in most cases, but in some it will become immediately apparent on smiling and speaking that a mistake has been made and too much tooth is showing. To satisfy all cases a more thoughtful approach is required, bearing in mind that a recent survey of complete denture patients has shown that more maxillary tooth was visible than in a population of dentate subjects.[4] The implication is that dentists tend to choose for edentulous patients an anterior occlusal plane which is lower than in life and which results in greater visibility of the maxillary incisor teeth.

The amount of maxillary tooth visible in the mouth at rest or when smiling depends on the differential development and growth of the lips and jaws. When obliged to make a judgement in the absence of a previous denture or when the previous denture is badly worn, the clinician can assume that the jaws are normally developed and assess the proportionate size of the upper and lower lips. The lower third of an ideal face may be divided horizontally into thirds. The upper lip (extending from the base of the nose to the commissures of the lips) occupies the upper third, and the lower lip and chin (extending from the commissure of the lips to the lower border of the chin) occupies the remaining two thirds. This proportion is well known to artists and can be used by the clinician to achieve a harmonious tooth/lip relationship. If after measuring the upper lip with dividers it is found that with the patient at rest it is approximately 1/3 of the distance from the base of the nose to the base of the chin, then the maxillary wax rim can be trimmed level with the lower border of the upper lip. When the upper lip is disproportionately larger or smaller, either the level of the rim can be correspondingly raised or lowered until judged harmonious by the operator or alternatively the rim can be adjusted until the distance between the lower border of the nose and the edge of the rim is 1/3 of the height of the lower third of the face (Fig. 4.4A and B).

Minor changes in the relationship of the lip line to the natural teeth occur with age and can be allowed for at this stage. It is known that with greater age the muscle

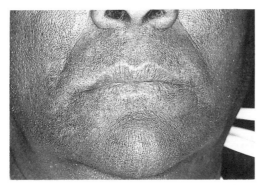

Fig. 4.4A Patient with disproportionately long upper lip who will prove a problem when siting the incisal plane.

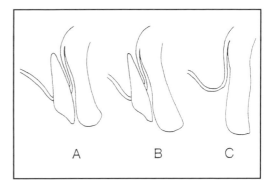

Fig. 4.5 Diagram of changes in lip form with age. A, young adult, B, elderly dentate patient with tooth attrition and longer lip due to loss of muscle tone. C, edentulous patient with collapsed lip.

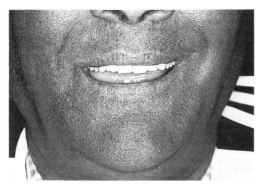

Fig. 4.4.B Best appearance is achieved with a high incisal plane. The raised, smiling lip now shows a normal amount of tooth.

tone of the upper lip decreases, the lip drooping and flattening to cover more of the anterior teeth (Fig. 4.5). The change is made a little more marked by attrition of the incisal edges of the anterior teeth. Changes of 1–2 mm are needed. To allow for the effect the level of the wax rims is raised 1–2 mm above the ideal position.

An alternative approach, which can be used as a confirmatory exercise, is to make adjustments of the wax in relationship to the smiling lip line of the upper lip. Best appearance is provided when 3–5 mm of upper tooth is exposed when the patient smiles, and this can be repro-

duced by trimming the upper rim to a mark made 3–5 mm below the smile line, raising or lowering a millimetre or so to correspond to an older or younger age group. First, however, check that the upper lip does rise on smiling. About a third of patients show little or no vertical movement of the upper lip and application of the rule then gives a toothy appearance at rest.

If the lip proportions are normal but the maxillary alveolus is well developed a large amount of maxillary tooth will be exposed on parting the lips. This is especially so if the maxillary alveolus is enlarged to the extent that it is visible on smiling (Fig. 4.6). Not only will a greater than normal amount of maxillary tooth be visible, but patients must be warned that without surgery it will be impossible to prevent the denture-base being visible when they smile.

A patient with a shorter than average upper lip or a prominent maxillary alveolus can be a problem if they ask for anterior teeth of a specific, normal size but expect only an average amount to show on smiling. The requested teeth can be provided but can be incorporated in the set-up only by lowering the occlusal

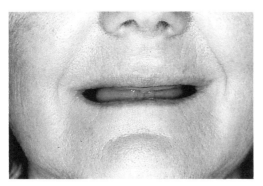

Fig. 4.6 The enlarged maxillary alveolus is visible on smiling. The patient will be dissatisfied with her appearance unless she is willing to accept that the denture base will also be visible on smiling.

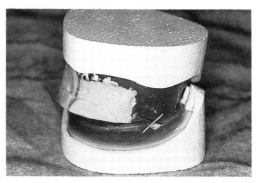

Fig. 4.7 Completed lip index showing the functional site of the maxillary teeth.

plane so that more tooth than normal is visible and so reproducing the patient's likely appearance before their teeth were lost. In the absence of surgery, success will depend on the operator's ability to persuade the patient to be satisfied with the original appearance. Without this compromise successful aesthetics is impossible.

For most patients with symmetrical faces the centre line of the face is easily identified and marked on the wax rim. When the patient's face lacks symmetry it is easier to fix the centre line according to pre-existing anatomical landmarks rather than from a general impression. The mean positions of the palatine papilla, upper labial fraenum and mid palatine suture are all within 1 mm of the midline tubercle of the upper lip,[5] but inherent biological variation means that it is best not to rely too heavily on a single landmark.

Lip index

As discussed in Chapter 2, there are techniques for recording the neutral zone which can be of use when biometric markers are inappropriate for identifying

the most stable position for the artificial teeth. A variation on the technique has been described[6] which serves to identify a position of stability for the anterior teeth only and is useful when treating patients who show marked muscle activity during function. The technique is used after the rims have been adjusted to give the required tooth visibility and are in even contact at the correct occlusal face height. The wax rim in the anterior region is removed from the maxillary block and the space is filled with a stiff mix of alginate. A coating of adhesive is needed to retain the alginate to the base. Replacing the block, the alginate is allowed to set while the patient protrudes their tongue slightly. After marking a centre line, the maxillary block is removed and the alginate trimmed to the vertical height of the remainder of the rim, then replaced and the blocks sealed in the retruded contact position (Fig.4.7). The process can be extended to include a record of the lower lip, when the lips are kept together and the patient makes swallowing movements. The technician casts a plaster matrix to the labial face of the block and uses it to ensure that the site of the anterior teeth conforms to the lip index.

Jaw relations

Establishing the correct jaw relationships is the most important clinical stage in the process of complete denture construction, and errors at this point are the most frequent cause of referral for specialist opinion following patient dissatisfaction with prosthodontic treatment.[7] If an unnoticed error has been made in recording the jaw relationships the subsequent intractable discomfort and instability can lead to complete loss of patient confidence.

Errors are easily made. The most obvious inaccuracy arises because the registration blocks are unstable or ill fitting. For those occasions when poor retention is noticed at the registration stage a proprietary powder denture fixative will suffice to retain the bases adequately. All traces of fixatives are to be removed from the base before returning the work to the technician otherwise dried fixative will prevent accurate relocation of the registration block on the working model.

Inaccuracies also arise due to restrictions in the methodology. The clinician is dealing with a human being and must use fairly simple measuring devices. Complex, accurate devices are available but involve expenditure of time or degrees of discomfort which would be unacceptable. There is also, as with all biological processes, the problem of normal variation and the clinician must have a clear idea of the normal range to ensure that his patients are not required to conform to an inappropriate model.

Vertical jaw relations

The basic intermaxillary relationship in the vertical plane is the rest or postural position. This is defined as the relationship between the maxilla and the mandible when the patient is seated, erect and dible when the patient is seated, erect and at rest. There, the jaws are uninfluenced by teeth or cuspal interferences and it is reasonable to assume that the relationship is constant whether the subject is dentate or edentulous. In the rest position the maxillary and mandibular teeth of the dentate patient are separated by a space, the interocclusal space. It is assumed that the relationship between the maxilla and mandible, and hence the size of the interocclusal space, is determined by the state of tone of the elevator and depressor muscles of the mandible, and this appears to have been confirmed by finding that the relationship is affected by head posture and the degree of flexion of the cervical vertebrae.[8] If, then, with the head in a standard posture and the patient relaxed, the vertical height of the lower part of the face is measured between two suitably sited arbitrary points, the resulting measurement is termed the rest face height.

Although the rest positions in the dentate and edentulous patient are analogous to one another and each is constant over relatively long periods of time it must not be assumed that they are unchanging. The transition from the dentate to the edentulous state is associated with a reduction in face height,[9] and it is likely that the edentulous patient suffers a gradual reduction in face height throughout life as a consequence of alveolar resorption, and despite regular prosthodontic efforts to maintain the *status quo*.

When the teeth are brought into maximal occlusion or maximal intercuspation the new relationship between the maxilla and the mandible is called the intercuspal or tooth position. The new face height is called the occlusal face height and, if measured between the previously established arbitrary points, will be found to be less than the rest face height by the size of the interocclusal space.

If these relationships are transferred to

the edentulous patient it will be seen that an intermaxillary relationship has to be recorded corresponding to the intercuspal position, so that the artificial teeth can be set up at the correct vertical jaw relationship. One way to do this is first to establish the rest position and measure the rest face height. If with the record blocks in place and in occlusion the face height is less than the rest face height by the extent of a previously decided interocclusal space the occlusal vertical jaw relationship will be correct. In dentate individuals the interocclusal space has a vertical range of 2–9 mm in the region of the anterior teeth. Clinical experience shows that complete dentures will function satisfactorily if an interocclusal space is chosen within the range of 2–5 mm. While most patients will be happy with an interocclusal space at the lower end of this range, it is best to use the upper end, even if only temporarily, if there are previous marked signs of overclosure. This can be manifested as extreme degrees of attrition of the artificial teeth or if there is an obvious compression of the lips with loss of visible vermilion border.

In the past a number of techniques have been suggested for measuring the vertical jaw relationship, but many have proved impracticable. Some 50 years ago Boos[10] claimed that by use of intra-oral strain gauges a reproducible maximum biting force could be measured at a degree of jaw opening thought to be equivalent to the occlusal face height. It was postulated that at this face height the muscles were in their most efficient state of extension and mastication would be most comfortable. While the technique is of interest to researchers it is difficult to imagine how it can be applied economically to clinical practice. The same criticism can also be levelled at techniques which seek to establish vertical jaw relationships at points of minimum muscle activity by means of electromyography. An interesting alternative technique for establishing the face height involved making accurately fitting bases and separating them by a screw-jack. Different degrees of jaw separation can be achieved by altering the screw-jack height and at each position the patient assesses their degree of comfort. The most comfortable degree of opening is claimed to coincide with the correct occlusal face height. This technique too has failed to make any impact in other than research circles.

Two or three techniques for measuring the vertical face height are in common clinical use. The first involves the use of dividers and can be used for all patients except those with beards. Small triangles of adhesive tape are placed on the tip of the patient's nose and most prominent part of their chin, and marked with ink dots. The vertical distance is first measured between these two points with the patient sitting, head erect in the chair. In order to ensure reproducibility of the position the patient must be relaxed, and it is best if the patient wears the set of dentures to which he is accustomed (or at least the mandibular denture if an error of excess face height is suspected). Every attempt is made to achieve a tranquil atmosphere by the elimination of noisy distractions and reassuring the patient by adopting an unhurried, non-authoritative manner. To further permit the musculo-skeletal relationships to be consistent for this and later visits, it is best to standardize the position of the head by ensuring that one of the fixed planes (most conveniently the Frankfort plane or alternatively the ala/tragus line) is horizontal.

After adopting the above precautions most patients allow their mandible to enter the rest position if they are asked first to lick their lips and then relax. Patients who are more tense are asked to open and close their mouths widely for a short while to fatigue the extensor muscles and then close until their lips come into relaxed contact. Whichever method is employed, dividers are used to measure the distance between the two marked points, which is recorded. After removing any dentures the record blocks are inserted, the patient asked to close, and the distance between the two points measured again. If the occlusal face height is correct the latter measurement should be 2–5 mm less than the former.

With this technique the common source of error is movement of the soft tissues over the chin. If the occlusal face height is excessive some patients will attempt to achieve lip contact by contraction of the circum-oral musculature. The skin surface then moves vertically in relationship to the underlying bone and an inaccurate measurement is made. Care must be taken to observe the action of the associated facial muscles during the procedure and to adjust the record blocks further if any skin movement is visible. The commonest movement is caused by contraction of the mentalis muscles and is visible as dimpling of the skin over the chin and elimination of the groove at the base of the lip (Fig. 4.8).

The second technique involves use of a Willis gauge. This device was once intended to measure the face height by a method popular before the concepts of rest and occlusal face height were confirmed. In the original technique the vertical distance between the commissures of the eyes and the mouth was compared to the vertical distance between the base of the nose and chin. If the distances were the same then it was assumed that the face height was correct because the facial proportions conformed not only to a predetermined mean, but satisfied a basic artistic harmony.

By rotating the sliding arm through

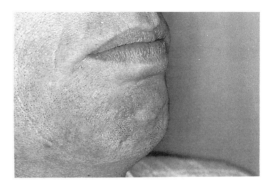

Fig. 4.8 The mentalis muscle is being contracted in an attempt to achieve lip contact when face height is excessive.

180° the device can be used in a more scientific way. Using the same methods as before the patient is encouraged to enter the rest position and the gauge placed on the face with the upper fixed arm fitting in the angle between the columella of the nose and the philtrum of the lip. The lower moveable arm is now raised to touch the lower border of the chin and the distance (the rest face height) measured and recorded. This is repeated with the record blocks in occlusion. The occlusal face height is now recorded and compared with the previous rest face height. The errors in this method are obvious. The upper and lower angles between the arms and body of the gauge rarely correspond to those between the columella and the philtrum and between the anterior and inferior surfaces of the chin. Reproducibility is therefore difficult to achieve between operators. Further, the contact of the device with the patient is over soft tissue and the measurements will vary according to the degree of pressure and the ability of the operator to detect soft tissue distortion. Nevertheless, the method is reputed to be accurate in experienced hands and high degrees of intra-operator (but not inter-operator) consistency have been claimed.[11]

Inevitably all methods in which measurements are made from superficial facial markers have a degree of inaccuracy, some investigators finding their use successful in only 2/3 of patients.[12] An alternative technique is one which while not quantitative, has many clinical advocates, and involves measuring the closest speaking distance. The method involves reducing the face height until the patient can pronounce "s" sounds comfortably and distinctly without there being interference between the rims. At this point an interocclusal space should be present. In dentate subjects the interocclusal or freeway space between the opposing teeth at rest does not have the same magnitude as the equivalent space between the opposing teeth at the closest speaking distance (it is usually greater) but in the edentulous subject the two can be assumed to be the same. The technique has the advantage that it does not involve measuring a rest position and it has been claimed to be less sensitive to changes in patient posture than use of dividers or Willis gauge.[13] It is difficult to apply with confidence unless the wax rims are reduced bucco-lingually to a thickness corresponding to the natural teeth so as to avoid interference with the tongue. Indeed, until experience is gained, it might be better to use the technique only at the try-in stage and then as confirmation of quantitative methods.

Although it is unwise to use the method of closest speaking distance on every occasion as the sole guide for establishing the occlusal face height, it can be very useful in those cases where prolonged wear of an ill-fitting denture by an elderly patient has taken place. The resulting gross over-closure makes it difficult to establish a jaw relationship which not only restores some of the lost face height but can be tolerated by the patient. Quantitative techniques, if rigorously applied, tend to increase the face height drastically and overstress patients' capacities to adapt. The method of closest speaking distance is also of use when establishing the occlusal face height for patients with a marked class III jaw relationship. This is often associated with a large gonial angle and excessive length of the lower third of the face—sometimes also with an anterior open bite. In such circumstances a technique which depends on functional relationships is more likely to restore the natural proportions.

Horizontal jaw relations

The presence of natural teeth allows two reproducible positions of occlusal contact to be identified, the intercuspal position in which maximal occlusal contact occurs and into which the jaws are guided on firm closure, by the cuspal inclines, and the retruded contact position which is reached when contact occurs between the teeth, with the condyles of the mandible in the retruded position in the glenoid fossae. In clinical practice the condyles can be made to enter the latter position either under the influence of physical pressure on the mandible by the operator or by his direction and encouragement of the patient. The retruded contact position in dentate subjects is not necessarily coincident with the intercuspal position and is usually reached after displacement of the mandible 1 or 2 mm further distally.

The cuspal inclines of natural teeth provide guidance for the mandible to pass into the intercuspal position. In the absence of the natural teeth only one reproducible contact position can be identified for the rims at the registration stage. This is the retruded position, with the mandible being guided into it by the help of the operator. Either physical pressure or verbal encouragement can be used, the mandible being a little further distal when using the former method on a relaxed patient than when using the latter. The position is consistent and clinical experience has shown that despite there being a discrepancy between the intercuspal and retruded contact positions in the dentate patient, successful complete dentures can be made by arranging for the patient's retruded contact position and the intercuspal position of the dentures to coincide. The high degree of success achieved demonstrates also the ability of the temporomandibular articulation to adapt to minor discrepancies in horizontal jaw relationships.

With wear of the cusps of denture teeth the intercuspal position may not be maintained and the patient can adopt a habitual position of occlusal contact. This can be very variable, especially in the elderly edentulous patient when attrition has entirely removed the cusps and hence all restraining influence of the artificial teeth is lost. If the position is tenaciously adhered to by an elderly patient it will interfere with the search for a reproducible position of retruded contact. When associated also with a degree of overclosure the mandible may pass into a habitual contact position with a considerable anterior displacement. Such positions of occlusal contact, although obviously pathological, when associated with overclosure may be very difficult to correct and if diagnosed at the assessment stage, attempts should be made to increase the face height by occlusal pivots or additions of resin to the lower occlusal surface. Even then replacement dentures may have to allow for an abnormal range of jaw movements by incorporating flat cusped teeth.

When even contact of the registration blocks has been produced at the correct occlusal face height several techniques are available for encouraging the condyles to pass into their retruded position in the glenoid fossae and recording the correct horizontal jaw relationship. Simple methods should be applied first. The patient is asked to relax and place the tip of his tongue as far distally on the soft palate as he can comfortably reach, while at the same time gently occluding the registration blocks. Functional traction is thus applied to the mandible via the insertion of the genio-glossus muscle. Confirmation that the condyles are in the correct site can be made by placing the tips of the index fingers over the glenoid fossae, immediately anterior to the tragus of the ear, and palpating their movements. If movement of the condyles back into the retruded site is not detected, repeating the movements a few times usually produces increasing degrees of success until the operator is confident that the true retruded position has been reached.

In some cases where bizarre habitual positions of closure have been adopted, further efforts are required. The patient can be encouraged to open and close his mouth widely for a few minutes to tire the muscles of mastication before the above manoeuvre is repeated. When the major opening and closing muscles, including the lateral pterygoids, are tired there is less likelihood of a protrusive position being adopted.

Once the patient has closed into the retruded contact position the blocks are located securely together. The simplest method is to use staples. If the operator is confident that the patient will close on command into the retruded position a staple can first be placed, points vertical, on each side in softened grooves cut in the lower rim (Fig. 4.9). The tips of these staples impale the maxillary block on

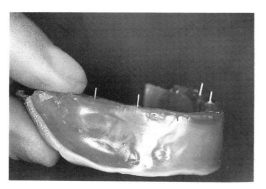

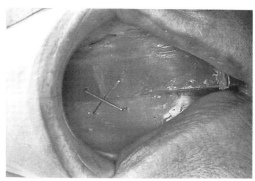

Fig. 4.9 Staples are placed vertically in the mandibular block to act as location aids.

Fig. 4.10 The registration blocks are finally located by staples placed buccally.

occlusion and ensure security of location. Two further staples are now pushed into the rims on each side, cross-wise (Fig. 4.10). After removing the united blocks from the mouth the rims are permanently sealed together on the lingual side with a hot knife.

Alternative location techniques require a little more expertise. If the patient can be trusted to remain for a short while in the retruded position, plaster or zinc-oxide/eugenol impression paste can be used as location materials. After cutting notches in the rims opposite one another in the premolar region, plaster or zinc-oxide impression paste is placed on the mandibular block and the patient asked to occlude and remain in that position until it has set. In an even simpler method, a shallow notch can be cut in the maxillary rim on both sides in the premolar region. After smearing a thin layer of petroleum jelly on the notches to act as a separating medium and building a mound of softened wax on the mandibular block, the patient closes into retruded contact which is maintained until the wax has set. The blocks can then be removed, cooled, separated and the retruded contact position confirmed by repetition. When the operator is sure that the blocks are correctly related they can

be sealed permanently, out of the mouth, with a hot knife.

When an abnormal position of occlusal contact exists it is very difficult to persuade patients to adopt the retruded contact position, and the method of using a gothic arch or arrow-head tracing can be useful. This method imposes lateral stresses on the blocks and for maximum accuracy not only must the bases fit the denture-bearing surface accurately but the ridges should be sufficiently well developed to give lateral stability. If there is doubt as to whether the ridges are well enough developed, then when it is thought an arrow-head tracing is going to be necessary it is best to anticipate the course of action and further ensure that retention is maximal by arranging for the wax rims to be made on permanent acrylic bases.

After adjusting the maxillary block to record the occlusal plane and soft tissue support, the bulk of the mandibular block is removed. An adjustable pointer is attached to the maxillary block and a scribing plate attached to the mandibular. The pointer is adjusted until the face height is correct. A range of anterior, posterior and lateral mandibular movements are made to check that there is no interference between the blocks. After coating the scribing plate with wax pencil, anterior–posterior movements of the mandible are made and when it is thought that sufficient retrusion has taken place, lateral movements are initiated. By careful guidance of the patient and repeated coating of the plate an entire arrow-head tracing will finally be made, the tracing representing the posterior V-shaped part of the envelope of movement of the mandible in the horizontal plane. A perforated acrylic disc is sealed with sticky wax to the scribing plate — the perforation superimposed over the apex of the arrow head. The assembly is replaced in the mouth and with slight encouragement the patient will permit the tip of the pointer to enter the perforation in the acrylic disc. The blocks are sealed together in this position by means of impression plaster placed in the pre-molar regions (Fig. 4.11).

Whichever technique is used, when the retruded contact position has been recorded the working models are related to one another via the record blocks, and it is here that a common error can lead to a mistake in the jaw relations. Care must be taken to ensure that the models do not contact each other in the hamular notch/retromolar pad region. If contact does occur the models must be carefully trimmed to eliminate the contact but without damaging the denture-bearing area. To leave the checking of this point to the technician is an undergraduate type of error which leads only to recriminations at a later date when the try-in is found to be faulty.

Articulators and facebows

The subject of articulators in complete denture prosthodontics is controversial. An articulator reproduces extra-orally the mandible, maxilla and temporo-mandibular joint relationships that have

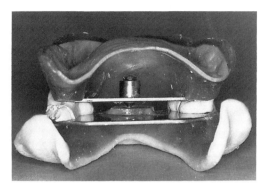

Fig. 4.11 Registration of antero-posterior jaw relation by use of arrow-head tracing. The assembly is viewed from behind to show components.

been recorded in the mouth at the registration stage. It serves to permit reproduction of mandibular movements and, in complete denture prosthodontics, the setting of the teeth in positions which allow the maxillary and mandibular dentures to provide mutual occlusal support. In use it is often helped by a transfer face bow, an auxiliary device which acts to transfer from the patient the relationship between the maxilla and condyles to those points on the articulator which act as analogues of the condylar heads. To perform this auxiliary function in three dimensional space it also records the position of another reference anatomical landmark which is reproduced on the articulator (usually the Frankfort or similar standard plane). More complex articulators allow dynamic intermaxillary relationships to be recorded by means of pantographic recordings.

A second type of facebow — a kinematic facebow — performs a related function. It is attached to the mandible, and includes a pointer for locating the precise hinge axis of the condylar head. It normally achieves secure attachment to the mandible via the standing teeth and for this reason is not often used for complete dentures.

Depending on the complexity of the articulator two degrees of functional occlusal contact between the opposing teeth of complete dentures are possible. The first is balanced occlusion in which a minimum of three point bilateral supporting contact occurs between the maxillary and mandibular teeth in the intercuspal position, and ideally in which all teeth have supporting contact. Because there is bilateral contact the dentures are stabilized by occlusal pressure in the retruded contact position but unless balanced articulation also exists occlusal stability is lost once any mandibular excursion from the intercuspal is initiated.

Balanced articulation is a more complex functional occlusal contact, where a minimum of three-point bilateral contact (and preferably multiple contacts) is present between the opposing teeth at all times in lateral and protrusive excursions. Its advantages are obvious. Patients' masticatory and non-masticatory contacts do not always occur in the intercuspal position, and when balanced articulation is present even eccentric contacts will have a stabilizing effect.

In complete denture prosthodontics the prime purpose of the articulator is therefore to allow the technician to set the artificial teeth in balanced articulation and enhance stability by permitting bilateral occlusal support when the dentures are in contact in both the intercuspal position and in lateral and protrusive excursions. On purely functional grounds it is debatable whether occlusal balance is relevant during mastication, because the presence of food in the mouth prevents the opposing occlusal surfaces contacting unless the food is soft enough to allow complete penetration of the bolus, and if the food is already of this consistency comminution is unnecessary. Nevertheless, no matter what its consistency, chewing food appears to be a pleasant occupation and it would be foolish to deny our patients any opportunity of stabilizing their dentures when indulging in this minor consolation.

By helping to provide stability during non-masticatory contacts the need for occlusal balance is more obvious. Dentures remain well retained so long as the integrity of the saliva layer between the denture-base and the supporting soft tissues is maintained. The thixotropic nature of saliva means that when displacing forces are minimal and low shear stresses are applied, it acts as a gel and allows dentures to maintain their position. However, the constant movements of the facial musculature during talking cause sufficient stress to shear the saliva layer and gradually displace the dentures unless they are deliberately reseated at intervals by occlusal contact. In the absence of balancing bilateral occlusal contacts, uniform reseating would not always take place and the dentures might have to be reseated in some other, less socially acceptable, way. Involuntary occlusal contacts also occur during swallowing. While in the absence of balancing bilateral occlusal contacts the swallowing contacts would tend to displace complete dentures; when present they enhance stability.

Articulators may be classified into Arcon type, where the condylar guidance is integral with the upper member, and non-Arcon type in which it is part of the lower member. Such differences are purely of design and on functional grounds, three types of articulator may be defined and are in common use. The first is the hinge articulator which reproduces only the hinge movements of the mandible in the glenoid fossa. The opposing artificial teeth can be set up to occlude in one position only and balancing occlusion of the teeth only follows hinge closure of the mandible into the intercuspal position. It is impossible to provide balance in lateral excursions.

The average value articulator is more complex and permits lateral and hinge movements of the mandible, the movements of the condyles being governed by preset average condylar guidance angles, and anterior guidance being provided by a fixed incisal guidance plane. Some means is also provided for the maxilla to be located an average distance from the condyle analogues. Balanced articulation is possible to the extent that the patient's mandibular movements in life correspond to the average movements predetermined by the articulator settings.

The third type is the adjustable articulator, which has a variable potential for reproducing the actual functional movements of the patient's mandible. It can reproduce parameters such as condylar guidance angles, incisal guidance angles, immediate and delayed Bennett shift, and permit accurate siting of the mounted models in positions duplicating the relationships in life. The accuracy with which adjustable articulators can reproduce the occlusal parameters varies and to this extent they are subdivided into fully adjustable and partly adjustable. The difference is artificial, however, and no articulator can reproduce all mandibular movements; to this extent all adjustable articulators are partly adjustable.

To provide balanced articulation, artificial compensating curves are incorporated in the arrangement of the teeth so that they can be placed in natural looking positions and at the same time function effectively and provide occlusal support. The first of these is the antero-posterior compensating curve. The teeth of modern man usually show little wear and in the absence of a bruxing habit the original form of the incisors is maintained throughout life. Consequently, as the dentate mandible moves forwards in occlusion and the condyles move forwards across the anterior slopes of the glenoid fossae, the anterior segment of the mandible is stabilized by the guidance the mandibular incisors receive by maintaining contact with the lingual surfaces of the maxillary incisors, and the premolar and molar teeth pass out of contact. Lack of posterior contact would destabilize a complete denture and hence an antero-posterior compensating curve is incorporated in the occlusally contacting surfaces of the artificial dentition as a method of providing support for a denture during protrusive movements by maintaining sliding contact in the premolar and molar regions.

On an articulator, guidance equivalent to that of the glenoid fossae is provided posteriorly by the condylar guidance surfaces and anteriorly the guidance equivalent to that of the lingual surfaces of the maxillary incisors is reproduced by the incisal guidance table. The angles these make with the plane of orientation are called the condylar and incisal guidance angles. While on an adjustable articulator the condylar guidance angle may be altered to correspond with that of the patient, no such restraint is placed on the incisal guidance. Most authorities advise that for the sake of good appearance and ease of tooth arrangement the incisal guidance table is adjusted to provide an incisal guidance angle of approximately 10°. If cusped posterior teeth are set up with a normal bucco-lingual relationship, then because in protrusion the distal surfaces of cusps of the maxillary teeth must give support by maintaining contact with the mesio-lingual inclines of the cusps of the mandibular teeth, the working cusp angles (which are less than the actual cusp angles because the contacting maxillary cusps do not traverse directly up the mandibular cusps) of those teeth

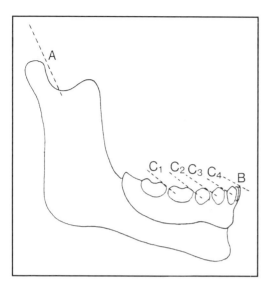

Fig. 4.12 The antero-posterior compensating curve produced by teeth tilted to form working cusp angles (C_{1-4}) integrated with incisal and condylar guidance angles. A, condylar guidance plane, B, incisal guidance plane.

near the incisal guidance table must approach the incisal guidance angle in magnitude. As teeth are sited more posteriorly the angle must increase in size to approach the condylar guidance angle.

The cusp angles of most cusped artificial teeth are approximately 20°. Consequently, a mandibular first premolar must be rotated in the sagittal plane to further decrease the working cusp angle. Mandibular teeth lying more posteriorly must be upright or be rotated the opposite way in order to modify the working cusp angle appropriately as it comes further under the influence of the condylar guidance angle which is approximately 40°. In order to ensure such an arrangement of the teeth and at the same time maintain a normal mesiodistal contact, the teeth are set in a compensating curve which is convex downwards (Fig. 4.12). To some extent the above explanation is a simplification and depends on the cusps of artificial teeth being manufac-

tured as precise, geometrical cones, and the inclines of these cones traversing up the inclines of opposing cones in mandibular protrusion. To this extent the explanation is only an approximation, but nevertheless valid in principle.

The lateral compensating curve may be explained in an analogous way, again for opposing teeth in the normal bucco-lingual relationship to one another. When the mandible translates laterally, rotating around one of the condyles, the denture must maintain bilateral contact as the translating condyle moves downwards and forwards. Viewing the movement in the coronal plane, on the rotating side the buccal slopes of the mandibular buccal cusps must maintain sliding contact with the lingual slopes of the maxillary buccal cusps, and on the translating side the lingual slopes of the mandibular buccal cusps must maintain contact with the buccal slopes of the maxillary lingual cusps. With the anatomical relationship of condyle and occlusal plane found in the human, this is impossible unless the occlusally contacting maxillary lingual surfaces are of different angles, those nearer the rotating condyle more approaching the horizontal. To bring this about using constant angle cusps and at the same time permit occlusal support during translation to either side, the tips of the cusps of the maxillary teeth are tilted buccally so artificially decreasing the angle of incline of the lingual slope of the buccal cusps and increasing the angle of the buccal slope of the lingual cusp (Fig. 4.13). The degree of tilting required to modify the angle, and hence the downward convexity of the curve, varies with antero-posterior position; more anterior teeth requiring less tilting as the influence of the downward movement of the translating condyle decreases.

Although the antero-posterior and lateral compensating curves are entirely

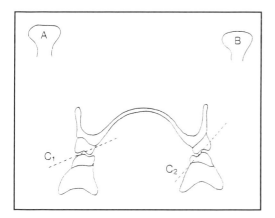

Fig. 4.13 A lateral compensating curve produced by teeth tilted to form working cusp angles ($C_{1,2}$) integrated with the lateral translation movements of the mandible. A, rotating condyle, B, translating condyle.

artificial and are needed to provide for dentures a bilateral occlusal support which natural teeth do not need, the inclinations they give to the artificial teeth resemble the inclinations which develop in the natural dentition. It is therefore possible to provide dentures with stability and natural appearance. However, to give more precise working balance several other factors must be included. In addition to the influence of the condylar and incisal guidance angles, the final geometry of the compensating curves and the precise degree of tilt of the teeth will have to be further modified by the influence of the immediate and delayed Bennett shift. Further, even assuming that no human error occurs and all parameters influencing occlusal function have been registered accurately, precise balance for a complete denture will still not be possible because the fully-adjustable type of articulator cannot reproduce the slight movements of the variably thick and variably visco-elastic mucoperiosteum beneath the denture under masticatory stresses; or the elastic

strain of the mandible as it bends medially and laterally under the influence of the muscles of mastication; or any elastic strain in the temporo-mandibular joints.

Adjustable articulators are expensive in terms of cost of purchase and time consumed, and clinicians may seek reasons to justify their use. The rationale for the use of articulators in complete denture prosthodontics can be summarized as follows. While many clinicians advocate complex articulators, and claim excellent results from their use, it has been difficult to confirm these results by clinical trial. To date, clinical trials comparing complete dentures with and without balanced articulation have failed to confirm an advantage for either when judged on the basis of patient satisfaction or pathological change[13] and it may be difficult to justify the use of an adjustable articulator on this basis. Clinical impressions of the superiority of adjustable articulators may be criticized as being more a consequence of the greater time and care that goes with their use rather than their intrinsic superiority.

Some might say that results like this point to the inadequacy of complex articulators, deny the possibility of ever recording all the factors needed to ensure balanced articulation, and point to the success of the vast majority of complete dentures made without the benefit of an adjustable articulator. Explanations for the lack of difference may be simple. Most dentures made on simple hinge and average value articulators are provided with acrylic teeth. While the strength of acrylic teeth has improved with the introduction of cross-linked resins, they are still susceptible to abrasion. Attrition of premature cusps may therefore convert an imbalanced occlusion into a model of occlusal efficiency during the first few weeks of denture wear and to a considerable extent remove differences between the two types of occlusion. Nevertheless, no trials to date have compared simple and complex articulators when used to treat problem cases, and the advantages of a more precise balanced articulation may be realized only when functional problems are exacerbated by a clinical difficulty. For this reason a technique for use of a popular adjustable articulator is included in the Appendix.

Alternative occlusal schemes

The stability of complete dentures depends to a considerable extent on the presence of well formed residual alveolar processes. In their presence natural looking teeth can be selected and arranged in ways which resemble life. When resorption is marked, stability decreases and alternative occlusal schemes have been suggested which promote stability by taking advantage of mechanical factors. Two are commonly encountered.

Flat-cusped (non-anatomic) teeth

At first sight the most acceptable solution to the lack of denture stability which results when the mandibular ridge is atrophic would appear to be an occlusal scheme based on the use of flat-cusped teeth. Lateral displacing forces arising from cuspal interference would then be minimized. Inevitably there are functional problems because in the absence of cusps which would help maintain balance in protrusive and lateral excursions, the anterior and lateral compensating curves have to be unacceptably steep. The usual solution is to set the premolars and first molars to a horizontal plane but to incline the second molars to form a balancing ramp which provides mutual posterior support in protrusion and to a limited extent in lateral excursions (Fig. 4.14).

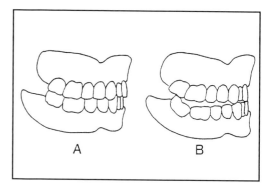

Fig. 4.14 An occlusal scheme for flat-cusped teeth. A, in retruded contact position. B, in protrusive contact.

While the modified occlusal scheme described above will enhance stability the lack of cusps diminishes the shearing component in mastication and patients may complain of inefficient chewing. The flat occlusal plane also has a poor appearance because it necessarily involves the anterior teeth and no vertical incisal overlap is possible.

Lingualized occlusion

With resorption of the mandibular alveolar process it is considered that if the mandibular occlusal contacts lie lingual to the residual ridge the mandibular denture will be more stable. In a lingualized occlusion only the lingual cusps of the maxillary teeth come into contact with the central fossae of the mandibular teeth and no contact occurs buccally, so moving the occlusal contact slightly lingually. Because only the maxillary cusps are involved in functional contact the occlusal arrangement for balance is simplified, the opposing teeth acting as a mortar and pestle. Such an arrangement can have its own problems however, because there is more need to maintain the integrity of the mandibular lingual cusps, and there is less latitude for their reduction to eliminate an unwanted undercut in the lingual polished surface.

Selection of teeth

This stage is particularly important in determining a patient's appearance. Most patients give little difficulty, but to aid understanding of problem cases it is useful to classify the three different types of good appearance which may be required to satisfy demanding patients. The first is the "natural look". This is the appearance which the dentist, with his training in dental anatomy and knowledge of the effect of the ageing process, believes is appropriate for the patient. The product of his expertise is a prosthesis, the teeth of which exhibit the attrition and discolouration complementary to the patient's age, and whose angulations and arrangements reflect the range of normal variation found in life. By use of the excellent materials available and his own informed observation the clinician can produce a replica of life. The patient suited to this appearance is well informed, intelligent, and conscious that their appearance should conform to that of their dentate peers. Typical members of this group are dentists and fellow professionals. When, after explanation and education a "normal" patient requires this appearance, the process of achieving it gives pleasure to all concerned.

As an alternative there is the "ideal look". Most patients are not acutely aware of the finer points of dental appearance and ask for teeth of a pleasing shade to be arranged in a harmonious fashion, reflecting the ideal appearance seen regularly in advertisements and colour magazines. Such a patient is best provided with teeth which harmonize with their features both in shade, size and shape. The arrangements which generally satisfy this group are those characteristic of youth and will work best with normal jaw relations. Problems arise when discrepancies in the patient's jaw relations necessitate, for denture stability, a tooth arrangement (generally an incisor relationship) which does not conform to their criteria for dental aesthetics. A patient with class III jaw relationship may have to accept instability of his maxillary denture if he wishes the maxillary incisors to be proclined into a normal relationship with the mandibular incisors, and a patient with a class II jaw relationship will find that to achieve a normal incisor relationship mandibular incisors have to be sited in a position where the mandibular denture is displaced by the lower lip.

Patients who appreciate the ideal look are concerned about their overall appearance but not interested in the minutiae. Such patients are numerous at all ages but are generally easily satisfied. Generally their main worry is that the tooth shade, size, and relationships should match their perception of the ideal and any reservations that they may have about other aspects they will bring up at the try-in stage when asked for their opinion.

Finally comes the "preferred appearance" group. Research has shown most patients not to be aware of slight difference in dental anatomy unless attention is drawn to them.[15] Rather, they prefer the regular (but not necessarily harmonious) arrangements achieved by orthodontists or request "small, white teeth". For one other section of this group the most important aspect is not the colour, size, and shape of the teeth but that the teeth should give the desired soft tissue support, and hence that they should be placed in the most favourable site. Such patients usually emphasize their particular need at the initial visit, which should prompt from the dentist an explanation of how their needs can only be met within the bounds of tissue tolerance. The final section of this group is those patients who have a preconceived idea of how their teeth were arranged in life. Much time may then have to be spent in providing teeth of exactly the right size, shade or mutual relationship, but without a precise match treatment is futile. Fortunately patients in this group are also easily identified. Either their previous dentures will display an obvious "fault"—a gold tooth or an unnatural form of diastema are common—or the patient will reveal their needs in profuse detail as they proceed with the selection process.

Selection of teeth for a patient is usually simple and problems are uncommon. When problems do occur they are notoriously difficult to diagnose and the repressed dissatisfaction of the patient is often not voiced until after they have been wearing the dentures for a while. Even then some patients are unwilling to be precise in their complaint lest they be considered oversolicitous about their appearance. For this reason the dissatisfaction may be expressed about other features of the denture design.

To avoid problems the clinician should be prepared to adopt a non-authoritative manner and if possible involve the patient directly in the decision making process—an approach which has been shown to achieve the best results.[16] In addition, the clinician should have available prepared material consisting of models and cuttings from magazines showing the range of tooth sizes, shapes and arrangements which occur in life. Photographs of previous successful cases are also useful. The clinician should also be prepared to explain the reasons for his actions as they arise and take a little time early on to identify which of the types of good appearance will best satisfy the patient's needs.

When, even after prompting, a patient will give no preference to help the operator in the choice of tooth size, shape or arrangement and it is envisaged that problems might occur, a useful strategem is to enlist the help of a relative. Many of the patients we see are elderly and may be accompanied by their children who provide physical or moral support, and are themselves dentate. Matching the shape and arrangement of a patient's teeth to those of a dutiful offspring can give pleasure to both and convince them of our desire to give the best possible result. The ploy should not be used if it is seen that the relationships between the two are less than good. The elderly can be difficult to please, and an old lady with time on her hands may not like a constant reminder of her real or imaginary domestic irritations.

Tooth material

The choice between acrylic and porcelain denture teeth is made on the basis of relative cost, appearance, mechanical strength and means of attachment. On the basis of price, acrylic always has an advantage and teeth of similar appearance are always more expensive when they are made of porcelain than when made from acrylic. However, even thought the best acrylic teeth have excellent appearance and are manufactured by the dough process from acrylic of two shades to simulate dentine and enamel, the finest appearance is achieved by porcelain. Minute imperfections and difference in colour can be added in the same way as for a porcelain veneer crown to produce a near perfect appearance. Although such characterization can be added to acrylic teeth after manufacture, acrylic is susceptible to abrasion and the permanence of such modification cannot be guaranteed.

Acrylic and procelain have very different mechanical properties. The main problem with acrylic is undoubtedly poor wear resistance. The development of cross-linked resins allowed acrylic teeth of greater toughness to be made, but unfortunately the resistance to abrasion, while increased, does not compare with that of porcelain. On the other hand, while procelain resists abrasion, it is brittle. Where acrylic resists impact due to its toughness, impact tends to cause brittle fracture of procelain. Fortunately the fracture predominently involves posterior teeth.

The physical properties of porcelain can work to its disadvantge and the resistance of porcelain to abrasion can be a problem. After 5 years, 32% of maxillary and 42% of mandibular dentures are claimed to require replacement.[17] To avoid risk of soft tissue damage complete dentures should be at least reviewed at a shorter interval, and some advise yearly review for fear early neoplastic change is missed.[18] Not unnaturally, the sight of intact porcelain teeth might encourage patients to imagine that the supporting tissues have remained unchanged and that no correction of the fitting surface is needed. The life of an ill-fitting prosthesis might then be unduly prolonged. When acrylic teeth are used, the obvious wear visible after a few years reminds patients that replacement is necessary before damage has been done to the soft tissues.

Although acrylic lacks the extreme hardness of porcelain, its lack of abrasion resistance can be helpful in other ways. The occlusal and incisal surfaces of teeth often need to be adjusted either during the setting up of the occlusion, or afterwards at the insertion stage if technical or clinical errors are present, or at the chairside if modifications are to be made to produce a lifelike appearance. The ease with which acrylic can be adjusted is then a very real advantage — especially in teaching hospitals.

Another less obvious advantage for acrylic is its mode of union with the denture base. Provided that the bonding surfaces are clean, then with teeth and base both being made of acrylic resin, a chemical union between the two is possible. With porcelain a chemical bond is impossible and instead retention is secured with pins or diatoric holes. Although the resulting mechanical retention is adequate for its purpose, the lack of bond means that the presence of the tooth makes an identation in the acrylic base which can be a source of weakness by acting as a point from which catastrophic crack growth can occur. Indeed it has been claimed that inadequate bonding of teeth is the most potent source of denture base fracture in use.[19]

Size of teeth

The time is long past when the only available denture-base material was Vulcanite and choosing tooth size was straightforward, being determined primarily by the need to choose teeth large enough to avoid any show of objectionably coloured denture base when the patient smiled. Today, the appearance of denture-base resins is excellent and tooth size is only a problem when the operator is faced with a patient demanding small, even teeth or some other combination which offends his aesthetic sense. Explanation and demonstration will usually persuade intelligent patients to a more conventional choice, but at times when faced with an adamant will, even the most persuasive clinicians must surrender — after all the patient is paying the bill.

When the patient does not demand a particular size of tooth the simplest approach is to choose the size of tooth according to the size of the patient, and dividers can be used to measure the total widths of the sets of six artificial anterior maxillary teeth supplied by the manufacturers. The sum total of the mean mesio-distal widths of the six maxillary anterior teeth of Western European populations is approximately 46 mm. To give to one's choice a harmony with the patient's size, a width of 46 mm can then be selected for a male patient of average build, 48 mm for a man of large build and 44 mm for a man of small build. Although there is no evidence that women's teeth are any smaller than men's, a woman's mean physical size is less and so to maintain harmony, for the corresponding three sizes of women the total mesio-distal widths of the selected teeth can be reduced by 2 mm.

When using this system patients are often surprised to see how large is the size of tooth which has been chosen for them. To confirm your choice it is wise to arrange for a few models of natural dentitions to be available so that a direct comparison can be made.

A related technique is one which seeks a correspondence in ratio between the average size of a tooth dimension and the average size of some anatomical feature. Popularly, a maxillary central incisor is chosen whose width corresponds to 1/12 of the width of the face (interzygomatic distance) or 1/20 of the height of the face (hairline to chin). Another popular method is to select a maxillary central incisor with a length equal to one quarter of the distance between the palatine papilla and the fovea palatini. This has the practical advantage of being easily and accurately measured on the working model with a pair of dividers. All depend on the assumption that the size corre-

sponding to the mean ratio in a population gives a harmonious appearance. With a little effort the reader can evolve his own system, taking one of the circum-oral features as the base. Then to the conviction that calculation brings, can be added the satisfaction of personal invention.

Alternatively (and especially for those frequent male cases where the hairline is indiscernible), the inter-alar width can be measured and used to predict the distance between the midpoints of the maxillary canines. The complication of this method is that the inter-alar width has been shown to equal the distance between the midpoints of the canines when the maxillary anterior teeth are set up to their natural curve. It can therefore be accurately applied only with either a certain amount of imagination or after making a provisional set-up. As a rider to this method, the golden ratio can be used to choose the relative size for the maxillary central and lateral incisors. It is believed that when viewed from the front the most harmonious relative widths are created when the central and lateral incisors are in the golden ratio to one another (approximately 5:3). The most harmonious width of the canine can be decided in the same way and its width (again when viewed from the front and correspondingly reduced) should be in the same decreasing golden ratio to the width of the lateral incisor.

The size of mandibular incisors is frequently misjudged by manufacturers and the mandibular teeth which are provided to correspond to the selected maxillary incisors are often much narrower than the sizes found in life. Without specific instructions, the technician will often prefer to choose smaller incisors which allow more latitude if the set-up proves difficult. The mean ratio of the width of the maxillary central incisor to the width of a mandibular incisor is 1:0.6, or alternatively the total width of the four mandibular incisors should be 2.4 times that of the maxillary central incisor. By prescribing for the technician incisor teeth corresponding to these ratios the aesthetic error of inharmoniously narrow mandibular incisors can be avoided.

Posterior teeth, too, are usually provided by the manufacturers in a range of sizes smaller than those in life. There are advantages in having small posterior teeth. In any one quadrant four posterior teeth of normal mesio-distal length will be difficult to set up in the often reduced amount of space available. On functional grounds too there are advantages in providing small teeth. Although it has been shown that the area of the masticatory surface is proportional to the efficiency of mastication, smaller occlusal areas impose lower pressures on the denture-bearing area and are likely to be more comfortable in function. Also, if the mandibular teeth are of normal bucco-lingual width the projection of the lingual cusps often creates an undercut which when engaged by the tongue destabilizes the denture. Fortunately, except when smiling very widely, variations in the bucco-lingual width of posterior teeth are invisible and on balance it is probably best to use posterior teeth narrower than those found in life. The only surfaces of posterior teeth which can be normally seen by an observer are the buccal surfaces of the maxillary premolars. Some manufacturers realize this and provide sets of posterior teeth which are of reduced size but in which the buccal surfaces of the premolars are of a length approaching that found in life.

Shape of tooth

The shape of teeth has fascinated dentists since the time it became possible to prod-uce aesthetic, functional dentures, and much effort has been expended in making the art of tooth-shape selection conform to some imagined law of harmony or proportion. Few of the schemes which have been proposed in the dental literature are based on scientific or anthropological evidence, but instead merely serve to give confirmation to an intuitive choice.

The earliest such proposal claimed that teeth were capable of expressing the temperament of the patient, and at the turn of the century dentists were invited to select teeth of shapes corresponding to the choleric, plethoric, sanguine or lymphatic temperaments that they encountered in their patients. Later Leon Williams suggested that maxillary incisor teeth should be chosen which had a shape corresponding to the inverted outline of the patient's face. Such a system had the advantage of simplicity and many manufacturers of artificial teeth have retained his classification of teeth into tapering, round and square shapes as the basis of their range of moulds. Most recently, Lee[20] has refined this system further by classifying the upright shape of the face according to the ratio that the widths of the forehead and the lower third of the face make to the interzygomatic distance, which serves as the standard. Patients with a forehead proportionately wider than their interzygomatic width would then have square teeth prescribed and patients with a proportionately wider upper lip would have tapering teeth prescribed.

An interesting and more rational method is to relate the shape of tooth to the shape of the maxillary ridge. This is not as arbitrary as it seems. Where a maxillary ridge is V-shaped and narrow, narrow tapering teeth are often the only type which will fit into the reduced space available. Correspondingly, by prescrib-

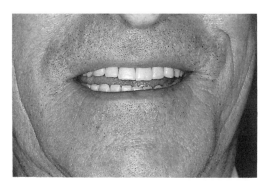

Fig. 4.15A Teeth modified to a "masculine" shape by alteration of their incisal edges.

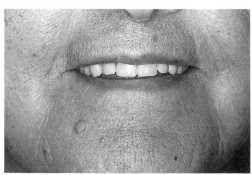

Fig. 4.15B The same mould teeth as before but modified this time to give a "feminine" appearance.

ing broad square teeth for a patient with a square ridge form, it is technically easier to fit six such anterior teeth into the inter-canine space. Less rationally, the convexity of the labial surfaces of the incisors has been related to the general degree of convexity of the patient's face in profile. While, as might be expected, no correlation occurs in life, one can imagine that the general facial harmony of a patient with a convex profile would be complemented by convex teeth. To complete such a facial harmony, just as it has been suggested that the golden ratio can be used in the selection of tooth size, it can also be used to select tooth shape. Hence for maximum harmony the height: width ratio of anterior teeth should be close to the golden ratio of 5:3.

Another popular method for selection of tooth shape is that advised by Frush and Fisher in the 1950s.[21] They hypothesized that men, who were imagined as having square, angular physical forms, should be provided with square, angular teeth in order to produce harmony of shape. On the other hand women, who were seen as curved, rounded creatures, should be provided with teeth of a curved and rounded form. Clinicians were therefore advised to modify the shape of

selected teeth to correspond with the patient's sex. While there is no actual relationship between sex and tooth shape, this method can produce some remarkably sympathetic results, especially when —as often occurs—the hypothesized differences in physical form are reflected in the shape of the patient's face (Fig. 4.15A and B).

No discussion of tooth shape would be complete without a mention of attrition. Most patients for whom we make complete dentures are elderly and if they had natural teeth they would show evidence of wear. A sure sign of the presence of a denture, despite careful choice of materials, is lack of attrition. To ensure that a clinician's work has the stamp of reality it is necessary to persuade patients that some evidence of attrition must be incorporated. Removal of 1–2 mm from the incisal edge of each incisor tooth (including the mandibular incisors) is generally enough. Care should be taken when adjusting the maxillary teeth to produce not a straight line of wear but a series of slightly angled facets, each articulating with the mandibular incisal edges (Fig. 4.16). While facets resembling attrition can be cut in the selected incisor teeth by the clinician and later set up by the tech-

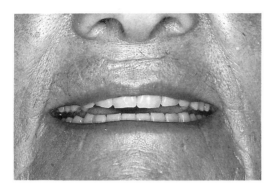

Fig. 4.16 An example of simulated attrition.

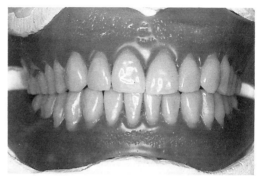

Fig. 4.17 A try-in showing simulated root exposure.

nician, most clinicians prefer to leave any modification to the try-in stage and then ask the technician to bring the incisal edges of the mandibular anterior teeth into occlusion by readjustment of the set-up. Care has to be taken that when adjusting incisal edges that the cut is inclined upwards as it passes from buccal to lingual—as occurs in life.

At the same time as signs of attrition are prescribed it may be advisable to give instructions to the technician if another sign of ageing, namely root exposure and overeruption, is to be introduced. While it is possible to produce this appearance at the try-in stage by cutting back the wax at the cervical margin of selected teeth (Fig. 4.17), there may be problems if the alveolar processes are well developed. Unless prior warning is given that simulated root exposure will be needed, the technician may have altered the cervical margins of the incisor teeth to make them fit more easily into the restricted space available and limit the potential for producing the effect realistically.

When selecting the shape of teeth the busy clinician is more likely to be impressed by selection methods which are of practical benefit and are of proven worth in ensuring good appearance. In that case it is best to select teeth of a generally square/oval shape. Such teeth are easier to set up and modifications to the contact points, which are frequently needed to ensure functional occlusion, can be made without obvious alteration to the general shape. Further, square teeth have long contact points and even when the incisal edges have been reduced by simulating attrition, the contact point is low enough for a papilla to be represented without the acrylic "gingivae" having to fill a large interproximal space and give poor appearance by extending too far towards the incisal edge. If root exposure is also to be imitated, square teeth are essential, otherwise the artificial increase in clinical crown length produces such a deep interproximal space that appearance and hygiene both suffer.

Recent research into patient preference also supports a choice of square/oval teeth and implies that they are the shape to be selected for all cases. Trials were carried out of the preferences of patients and dentists. Basing their judgement on aesthetics, both groups made a selection from teeth of various shapes and both showed a preference for square or oval teeth rather than tapering teeth.[22] Even female patients made this choice without displaying the definite preference for round shapes which harmony might suggest are most appropriate. It could be that the aesthetic complement of round teeth with the female sex (as mentioned above) is one which exists only in the eyes of a male observer.

Artificial posterior teeth with an anatomy based on natural teeth are satisfactory in most cases, but when alveolar atrophy is marked a case can be made for non-anatomic posterior teeth without cusps. In an endeavour to provide an alternative way of cominuting food, manufacturers once provided posterior teeth with inverted cusps, namely geometrical grooves and slots cut in the occlusal surface, or even grooved metal occlusal surfaces. An easier way of making flat cusped teeth which will not cause instability of a denture by cuspal interference is to modify a normal denture tooth. The problems of articulation arising from such a choice have been dealt with earlier.

Shade of tooth

Because this book is principally concerned with clinical practice, a long digression on the physiology of colour perception is unwarranted. Briefly, manufacturers produce guides for the practitioner with two basic colours or hues, red and yellow, present in varying amounts or intensities. The value, or lightness or darkness, of the colour is a measure of the degree to which it reflects or absorbs light. Only the lower values are relevant to tooth selection. The tooth shades in the manufacturers' guides are therefore mixtures of low intensity hues, the grey shades being hues of such low intensity as to be imperceptible.

The problems that a dentist is likely to come across are three. There may be problems choosing the most appropriate

shades for the patient; there may be problems convincing the patient that your choice is correct; there may be problems ensuring that the selected teeth have the detail characteristics which satisfy the patient's needs for realism.

If at all possible, selection of the shade should take place in natural light—a north facing window is ideal. This is not always possible, some surgeries being entirely artifically lit. In the absence of a natural light, a light source with an emission spectrum resembling daylight gives best results. Most manufacturers provide a wide range of shades, and for complete denture prosthodontics where it is unnecessary to match shades with natural teeth, the process is straightforward. The first stage is to identify those hues which best suit the patient's complexion. Generally a fair complexion is best matched with a reddish hue, a swarthy complexion with a yellowish hue, and for the elderly a greyish hue is best. Having identified the correct hue, the set of six maxillary anterior teeth selected from the guide may be wetted and placed in the shadow of the upper lip while the patient observes the process with a large hand mirror. Rarely will more than two or three of the lighter (low value) shades be needed, although good patient management may require an explanation as to why the full range of hues and values is not being used.

If a male dentist has consistent difficulty with differentiating between hues the fault may be that he has inherited some degree of colour blindness. The condition, if identified, is most easily overcome by delegating the choice of shade to a female DSA. Women rarely suffer from this sex-linked disease and are usually more expert at colour matching by dint of past experience with selection of household fabrics and furnishings. Female patients are often very interested in this aspect of treatment and because they may suspect a male dentist to be less sympathetic to their needs, inclusion of the DSA in this aspect of the selection process has a positive effect on patient management.

A different problem to overcome when selecting tooth shades is conflict between the operator and the patient over the most appropriate shade. It is difficult for us to imagine a situation in which we ourselves would wish to have teeth of unnatural whiteness and we tend to assume that our patients have the same type of preferences. If our patients have been instructed in dental aesthetics this may well be the case, and little instruction is required for younger patients who have a high degree of dental awareness. Older patients are usually concerned with efficient, comfortable function and will often agree with us after a brief explanation. Some of our elderly patients, however, live in a society in which complete dentures are the norm and no stigma is attached to their use. Indeed, obviously new complete dentures imply a level of wealth high enough to afford them and they may rise in the esteem of their peers by being able to show them off. Should we diminish their pleasure by insisting that our choice is correct? What we lose in the opinion of their more perceptive friends we might gain by the communally-voiced praise of a satisfied patient. If we try too hard to convince such patients our enthusiasm can be counter-productive and the grudging agreement that is given at the try-in stage might turn to obdurate dissatisfaction in the face of family ridicule. Better to give patients what they want!

Despite being able to satisfy the patient with the correct shade, there remains the possibility that while generally correct the chosen tooth does not satisfy the patient's detailed demands for a life-like representation. Unless worn smooth by toothbrush abrasion, the labial surface of a natural tooth is not smooth but is composed of a series of plane surfaces. Each surface reflects light at a slightly different angle and produces variations in colour value. Manufacturers try to imitate this effect by modifying the surface of their teeth to a greater or lesser extent. When a patient asks for a greater amount of surface irregularity, extra facets can be cut vertically into the labial surface with a rubber wheel. Remember that only recently erupted teeth, which have yet to be worn by use, show well developed faceting and if the illusion of reality is to be preserved, reserve the effect for younger patients. Sharp instruments should never be used for faceting the tooth surface because they tend to score the surface, although very small stones and steel burs can be used to produce small defects and also to cut horizontal channels imitating the effect of perikymata.[23] Very careful polishing is then essential to avoid losing the characterization.

It is nowadays rare for patients to ask for gold inlays to be placed in their artificial teeth. On those occasions when it becomes necessary, a pinlay is the best choice. After taking a wax pattern of the prepared tooth, the inlay is cast and polished. The restoration is cemented in with composite resin after roughening the surfaces of the pins. Imitations of discoloured anterior composite restorations and more complex variations in shade can be introduced by means of proprietary staining kits, of which "Minute Stains" (George Taub Products, New Jersey) is the most popular. These are applied at the insertion stage. If introduced at the try-in stage they will be removed during the polishing process.

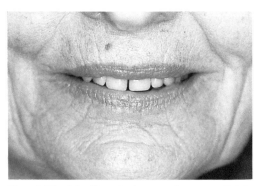

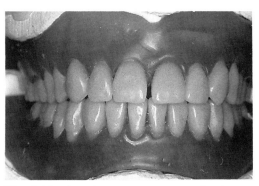

Fig. 4.18 Maxillary incisors set up parallel to the lower lip. The degree of harmony produced might be thought inappropriate for a patient of this age but is lessened by the presence of a central diastema.

Fig. 4.19 A try-in showing a correctly shaped central diastema.

Arrangement of teeth

The prescription for tooth arrangement may be complex and provides scope for skilful imitation of nature. Certain arrangements of teeth are characteristic of specific jaw relationships and can be prescribed if the patient conforms to that relationship and wishes to recapture the appearance of their natural teeth. Some patients who have a class II jaw relationship would once have had an Angles class II div ii incisor relationship, with overlapping of the disto-labial corners of the maxillary central incisors by the mesio-lingual corners of the lateral incisors. This can easily be recaptured in the artificial set-up, and gives a powerful illusion of reality, especially when provided for relatively young female patients, in whom it is hoped to enhance the appearance of femininity. Only in exceptional circumstances would an Angles class II div. i relationship be prescribed; not only does denture stability suffer but appearance is poor. Orthodontists derive a good proportion of their income from correcting such tooth arrangements.

The most well known way of providing a harmonious, attractive appearance for young female subjects is by setting the incisal tips of the maxillary incisor teeth parallel to the edge of the lower lip when they smile (Fig. 4.18). Too much emphasis of this arrangement in older subjects produces a disquieting effect, and if it is introduced into the tooth arrangment for a man, the feminine aspect is unduly emphasized. When an illusion of masculinity is to be provided it can be engineered by making the central incisors slightly more prominent than the lateral incisors. Such an illusion works best if also accompanied by attrition facets in the incisal edge. The effect can be further enhanced if it is associated with a reduced overjet or even edge-to-edge occlusion. Obviously this is easiest with patients whose jaw relationships verge on skeletal III.

An alternative means of emphasizing the masculinity or femininity of the tooth arrangement, and which can be used in conjunction with the above tooth arrangement, is to modify the angle of the maxillary canines. By inclining the tip of the canines lingually a more feminine appearance is produced, and a more

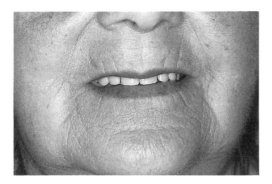

Fig. 4.20 Appearance for this patient is improved by the inclusion of diastemas and variations in tooth angulation.

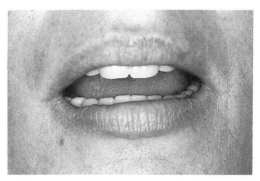

Fig. 4.21 By elongating the mandibular central incisors a more realistic appearance is achieved.

musculine appearance by inclining the tips of the canines buccally (Fig. 4.15B).

Whether or not to incorporate a diastema is a problem which can lead to dissatisfaction if not approached with care. The commonest type of diastema to be requested is one between the maxillary central incisors. Care has to be taken to ensure that diastemas can be kept clean. A diastema which is narrower at the incisal edge than the cervical margin is to be avoided, otherwise fibrous foods lodge in the space and are embarrassing to remove. By making the diastema wider at the incisal edge it becomes self-cleansing (Fig. 4.19). The effect of diastemas is to increase the life-like appearance, especially when they are also associated with variations in tooth angulation and attrition (Fig. 4.20).

The reverse of spacing—crowding— must be approached with caution. It is a simple irregularity to include but often causes difficulties because the lingual surfaces in contact with the tip of the tongue are irregular and a source of discomfort. The most acceptable crowding, and one which confers a great deal of reality on the tooth arrangement, is

crowding of the mandibular incisors. Crowding associated with retroclination of the mandibular lateral incisors is common and easily reproduced. However, for maximum life-like effect the retroclined incisors must be slightly elongated (Fig. 4.21).

References

1. Brook, I.M. and Lamb, D.J. A safe alternative to the gas flame. *Dental Practice* **26**:26, 1988
2. Watt, D.M. and Likeman, P.R. Morphological changes on the maxillary denture bearing area following extraction of teeth. *Br Dent J* **136**:225–235, 1974.
3. El-Gheriani, A.S., Davies, A.L. and Winstanley, R.B. The gothic arch tracing and the upper canine teeth as guides in the positioning of upper posterior teeth. *J Oral Rehabil* **16**:481–490, 1989.
4. Watson, R.M. and Bhatia, S.N. Tooth positions in the natural and complete artificial dentitions, with special reference to the incisor teeth: an interactive on-line computer analysis. *J Oral Rehabil* **16**:139–153, 1989.

5. Latta, G.H. The midline and its relation to anatomic landmarks in the edentulous patient. *J Prosthet Dent* **59**:681–683, 1988.

6. Anderson, J.N. and Storer, R. *Immediate and Replacement Dentures*. 3rd Edition. London: Blackwell Scientific Publications, pp 289–290, 1981.

7. Smith, J.P. and Hughes, D. A survey of referred patients experiencing problems with complete dentures. *J Prosthet Dent* **60**:583–586, 1988.

8. Murphy, W.M. Rest position of the mandible. *J Prosthet Dent* **17**:329–332, 1967.

9. Tallgren, A. The continuing reduction of the residual alveolar ridges in complete denture wearers. A mixed-longitudinal study covering 25 years. *J Prosthet Dent* **27**:120–132, 1972.

10. Boos, R.H. Intermaxillary relation established by power biting. *J Am Dent Assoc* **27**:1192–1199, 1940.

11. McMillan, D.R. and Imber, S. The accuracy of facial measurements using the Willis bite gauge. *Dent Pract* **18**:213–217, 1968.

12. Carrosa, S., Catapano, S., Scotti, R. and Pretti, G. The unreliability of facial measurements in the determination of the vertical dimension of occlusion in edentulous patients. *J Oral Rehabil* **17**:287–290, 1990.

13. Araki, N.G. and Araki, C.T. Head angulation and variations in the maxillomandibular relationship. Part I the effects on the vertical dimension of occlusion. *J Prosthet Dent* **58**:97–100, 1987.

14. Ellinger, C.W., Wesley, R.C., Abadi, B.J. and Armentrout, T.M. Patient response to variations in denture technique. Part VII twenty-year patient status. *J Prosthet Dent* **62**:45–48, 1989.

15. Marunick, M.T., Chamberlain, B.B. and Robinson, C.A. Denture aesthetics: an evaluation of laymen's preferences. *J Oral Rehabil* **10**:399–406, 1983.

16. Brigante, R.F. Patient assisted esthetics. *J Prosthet Dent* **46**:14–20, 1981.

17. Heath, J.R. Denture identification – a simple approach. *J. Oral Rehabil* **14**:147–163, 1981.

18. Brook, I.M. and Lamb, D.J. Surgical/ prosthetic problems of a large leaf fibroma. *Dental Update* **15**:126, 1988.

19. Lamb, D.J., Ellis, B. and van Noort, R. The fracture topography of acrylic dentures broken in service. *Biomaterials* **6**:110–112, 1984.

20. Lee, J.H. *Dental Aesthetics*. Bristol: Wright, 1962.

21. Frush, J.P. and Fisher, R.D. How dentogenic restorations interpret the sex factor. *J Prosthet Dent* **6**:160–172, 1956.

22. Brisman, A.S. Esthetics: a comparison of dentists' and patients' concepts. *J Am Dent Assoc* **100**:345–352, 1980.

23. Donahue, T.J. Facial characterization of anterior artificial teeth. *J Prosthet Dent* **49**:577–578, 1986.

Chapter 5

Try-in Stage

At the try-in visit we can judge the quality of our clinical work and the degree of communication that we have established with the patient and technician. Much time is involved with checking in an orderly routine that work has been performed according to prescription, and finally a number of associated procedures are carried out.

First, the jaw relations have to be checked and it is difficult to be certain that they are correct unless the bases for the try-in are retentive. Although the site of the artificial teeth will have been determined by the carved wax rims, minor changes in tooth position may be made when muscle interference is observed. If the appearance is not entirely satisfactory, chairside alterations to the site and shape of the teeth may be needed as well as modifications to the waxwork. Later, speech tests may be required to confirm that the teeth are in their correct functional position in the muscle matrix. Finally when all stages have been completed to everyone's satisfaction the post dam is cut in the appropriate place and instructions given to the technician either for any alterations which might be necessary for a retry, or for the technical stages to be completed and the denture processed in the selected denture base material.

Retention and stability of try-in

The choice of material for the base of the try-in is critical. Like the registration block, the try-in will be in the patient's mouth for several minutes and so the base must not only be of a material which is easily adapted to the working model by the technician in the laboratory but has to be resistant to distortion induced at mouth temperature. If permanent acrylic bases have not been made then shellac is the material of choice. Wax by itself softens too easily for clinical use.

It is impossible to perform a try-in confidently if the bases are poorly adapted and unretentive. Not only is it difficult to confirm the jaw relationships accurately, but speech tests give ambiguous results and the patient's confidence will be diminished, despite reassurance that retention will be improved at a later stage. If retention is poor due to the ridge form, good retention has to be ensured by means of a denture adhesive which acts by maintaining an intact, highly viscous, fluid layer between the base and the denture-bearing area.

All denture adhesives consist of a water soluble polymer, either natural or synthetic, usually polyethylene oxide, methyl cellulose or sodium carboxy-methyl cellulose. Powdered Karaya gum is no longer used; the pH of its solutions lies below the point at which enamel decalcifies[1], and manufacturers are no longer willing to market a product which although effective for complete dentures would have a destructive effect if inadvertently used to retain a loose partial denture or a complete denture opposed by natural teeth. The available types are produced in two formulations, those dispensed as liquids of various viscosities and those dispensed as powders. Both act in the same way and absorb moisture in the form of saliva to form a semi-solid gel on the surface of the denture or the base of the try-in. As far as the clinician is concerned, the essential difference between the two types is that the powder forms a viscous gel more rapidly than the liquid. Hence although the period of action of the liquid adhesive may be more prolonged, the powder form is to be preferred. Not only is its clinical effect more rapid, but when used with an ill-fitting base its gel-like structure is more suited to filling the often wide gap.

If denture adhesives are used to improve the retention of a try-in they must be completely removed afterwards, otherwise they will dry out to form a tough surface coating and make the try-in more difficult to replace accurately on the model. Removal of those adhesives containing a proportion of polyethylene oxide is a little more difficult. They produce excellent retention by forming a tougher, more elastic gel than those containing cellulose derivatives.

The modiolus is a fibrous knot lying in the cheek approximately 1 cm lateral to the commissure of the lip. Into it dehisce the risorius, the buccinator and most of the intrinsic and extrinsic muscles of the lip. During facial movements, but especially during smiling and mastication, it exerts considerable pressure medially. Its ability to destabilize a poorly retentive mandibular denture is great and it is customary to support the modiolus mainly by the buccal surfaces of the maxillary premolar teeth. In those cases where stability of the mandibular try-in is affected, an improvement can be made if the mandibular premolar teeth are repositioned a few millimetres more lingual than would be needed for a normal overjet in this region. The modiolus will then be supported principally by the premolars of the retentive maxillary denture and improved mutual stability results.

Confirmation of jaw relations

Small changes to the shape of the occlusal plane of the anterior teeth or modifications to their angulation can usually be made by alteration of tooth positions at the chairside. Similarly, small premature contacts or occlusal defects involving one tooth can be corrected by the operator, provided that it is customary to perform a check record at the final stage. Defects in the coincidence of retruded contact and intercuspal positions are more serious and if, after encouraging the patient to close in the retruded contact position, the teeth do not intercuspate correctly, or after inspection of the anterior teeth there is a discrepancy between the upper and lower centre lines not present when the try-in is mounted on the articulator, a re-registration must be made and instructions given for a re-try.

To re-register the jaw relations the mandibular posterior teeth are removed and replaced with wax rims which are softened and the retruded contact position re-recorded. After inspection of the indentations made in the wax rim by the opposing maxillary teeth, the width of the rim is reduced to the width of a tooth and surplus wax removed with a sharp knife from the occlusal surface until the indentation of the opposing teeth is just detectable. The wax surface is re-softened and the recording performed again. This serves to eliminate any wax that may be interfering with the opposing cusps and causing lateral or antero-posterior deviation. Only when the opposing cusps produce a complete but barely visible row of indentations can this be claimed with confidence. To prevent accidentally re-mounting in the same position, the work is returned to the technician after removing the lower model from the articulator.

A re-try also has to be made, but without a re-registration, if the centre lines have been misrecorded and are to be changed. The corrected position is marked on the teeth with a wax pencil. Inevitably the alteration will involve moving posterior teeth.

Appearance

A shade and mould of tooth will have been chosen at the registration stage and can now be checked for harmony with the patient's complexion and features, or at least that they fully satisfy the patient's wishes. The actual position for the teeth will have been determined by the technician working to the prescription of the carved wax rim and the tooth arrangement will be that which was requested. However, there is now further opportunity for improving the appearance of a sometimes lifeless arrangement of the teeth, by modifications to tooth positions which are difficult to convey by written prescription. Alternatively, it may be necessary to carry out any refinements to the appearance suggested by the patient. Needless, to say, any unasked for modifications should be made only when the patient agrees, and with a brief explanation most patients will appreciate the care that the operator is taking and approve enthusiastically.

As mentioned in the previous chapter, one of the better known ways of achieving a harmonious appearance is to parallel the incisal edges of the maxillary teeth with the lower lip—a relationship which commonly occurs in life. The arrangement sometimes occurs in the artificial dentition without being planned if the subject's posture is such that the anteriorly convex occlusal plane is below the observer's eye level, or when with the subject standing erect the occlusal plane tilts up posteriorly. However, in most cases it has to be produced artificially by first moving the central incisors down 1 mm or so and the lateral incisors in the same direction but to a lesser extent. Slight further modifications can be made to improve the final harmony of lip/tooth relationship either by further changes in tooth position or by adjusting the distal corners of the maxillary incisors with a stone to emphasize the curve. This modification of tooth arrangement works best with younger subjects because in real life the attrition that accompanies ageing tends to level out the incisal edges and in an elderly patient a curved arrangement of the maxillary incisors would be recognized as an anachronism. Any worries that the rearrangement of the incisors would lead to occlusal imbalance are usually unjustified if the overjet is of near normal magnitude. When after replacement on the articulator it is found that interference does take place, the incisal edges of the mandibular incisors are reduced into sliding contact.

Functioning natural teeth suffer from attrition, and unless signs of attrition are provided in the artificial dentition the teeth will appear obviously false. Ideally, attrition should be introduced by the

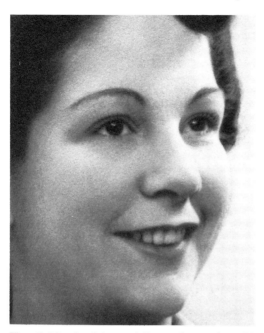

Fig. 5.1A A picture of the patient taken 50 years previously.

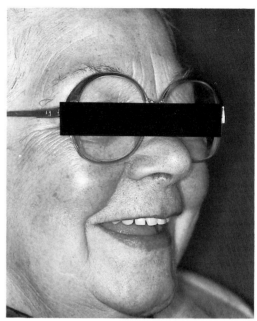

Fig. 5.1B The patient at present with complete dentures. Lip support has been maintained but the shapes of the teeth have been modified in a manner to be expected by the passage of time. Less tooth is shown, as would be expected at this age.

technician, while setting up the teeth to the operator's prescription, but if this has not been done the teeth can be modified now. With the wax try-in on the articulator, the maxillary incisal edge should be reduced by 1–2 mm to give the illusion of attrition. An obvious error is to cut the incisal facet horizontally across the incisal edge. Natural attrition does not occur in this way, and the cut surface should form a series of slightly angled facets. The mandibular teeth should not be neglected and incisal facets are also cut to articulate with those in the maxillary teeth. All facets should be angled upwards and backwards. To ensure that incisal contact occurs in protrusion the mandibular teeth can be raised slightly to produce protrusive contact.

After attrition facets have been cut, the extent to which the teeth show when smiling should be studied. Patients vary in the extent to which they reveal their maxillary anterior teeth when smiling. In some the action merely draws out the commissures laterally without significantly showing the teeth. In others the angles of the mouth are drawn up, the upper lip shortens and the gingival margins are visible as well as the entire labial surfaces of the anterior teeth. By measuring the length of the upper lip before and during smiling the shortening of the lip can be calculated and an estimate made of the likely amount of tooth that should be exposed. With this in mind the anterior segment of the occlusal plane can be altered to the patient's satisfaction. To help this process of siting the anterior plane correctly, photographs of patients before losing their teeth are invaluable, but when they are available account must be taken of the changes in lip posture and tooth shape that will have taken place during the intervening years (Fig. 5.1A and B).

At the same time distemas between the teeth can be incorporated or the appearance of crowding produced. Instructions are often given to the technician to produce this type of irregularity, but so personal is the patient's choice that the result is rarely completely satisfactory without some further adjustment according to the patient's precise specifications. The commonest request is for a space between the maxillary central incisors, but care has to be taken that the space provided is narrower at the cervical margin than the incisal edge, otherwise it will act as a food trap and be difficult to keep clean. A natural look can also be given by including spaces between the central and lateral incisors, and between the lateral incisors and canines. This must be done with care because if it is also associated with marked attrition the appearance of an "aged" dentition results (Fig. 5.1B).

When introduced at this stage, diastemas can cause technical problems. Unless the technician has already provided space for a diastema, the inclusion of one by the operator will lead to crowding of the remaining teeth. Sometimes this is slight and can be accommodated at the chairside by reducing the width of the canines without involving the posterior teeth. If substantial spacing is to be provided then the first premolars have to be removed and the technician instructed to provide a re-try for a final confirmation of the appearance.

Only a limited degree of crowding can be introduced before the irregularity that it produces soon makes it objectionable to the patient. A small amount can have a most pleasing effect, however, because the tilting that results breaks up any uni-

formity of angulation of the teeth and produces an "aesthetic" unevenness. In life, crowding is particularly common in the mandibular incisor region and can be simulated most realistically by retrolining the lateral incisors.

When creating a natural appearance it is possible to make use of the tendency for certain malocclusions to be associated with characteristic tooth arrangements. The commonest are the tooth arrangements associated with class II jaw relationships, in which the mandible is relatively distally placed in relationship to the maxilla. The degree to which the maxillary incisors are controlled by the upper lip determines two types of tooth arrangement. Where the maxillary central incisors escape from behind the lower lip, they are prominent and protrude beyond the mesial corners of the lateral incisors (Angle's class II div.i). Where the central incisors are well controlled by the lower lip they are retroclined and are themselves overlapped by the mesial corners of the lateral incisors (Angle's class II div. ii). Both types of malocclusion can be reproduced in moderation for relatively young patients (under the age of 50) with class II jaw relationships. They are then sometimes surprised to find the malocclusion of their natural teeth reproduced.

Practitioners who feel that the "masculinity" or "femininity" of a set-up ought to be emphasized can also employ this type of tooth modification. It is believed that the class II div. ii arrangement expresses a more female arrangement, especially if the tips of the canines are retroclined at the same time so that the cervical margins become more prominent. Conversely, the class II div. i is a more masculine arrangement. The feeling of masculinity can be additionally emphasized if the maxillary central incisors are more prominent than the lateral incisors and also if the canines are slightly longer and more prominent. A harder, masculine look is further emphasized if the set-up also incorporates a small amount of spacing and attrition. Care must be taken not to exaggerate the attrition and spacing otherwise, as mentioned above, an aged appearance results.

Finally, if the technician has not already done so, the shape and texture of the wax supporting the teeth can be altered to closely resemble the shape and texture of the surface of the alveolus. First, the topographical anatomy of the alveolus and marginal gingivae should be reproduced by addition and removal of wax, and a model of the natural dentition ought to be examined to achieve a clear picture of the ideal state. The labial and buccal surfaces of a complete denture should show the alveolar eminences over the "roots" of the teeth. These are most marked anteriorly and become less so in the premolar region. In the maxillary anterior region the canine eminence is most marked, with the central incisor less so and the lateral incisor often almost missing. In the mandible, again the canine eminence is the most marked with the incisor roots less prominent. Each alveolar eminence is at its maximum size near the gingival margin, tapering apically.

The natural healthy attached gingivae show stippling where collagen bundles tie down the mucoperiosteum to the underlying bone. Stippling is more pronounced in older patients and occurs in a band between the alveolar mucosa and the free gingival margin. Although the attached gingivae is not normally visible in life unless the patient has a high lip line, under these circumstances if surface stippling is reproduced in the acrylic of the base a most realistic appearance is created.

Stippling may be applied in two ways.

The simplest is by means of a toothbrush from which all expect a few terminal tufts of shortened bristles have been removed. By jabbing the surface of the wax with the tips of the bristles a pock-marked appearance is produced. Flaming the rough surface removes the grosser irregularities and a matt surface finish results which closely resembles natural stippling. The surface is finally polished with water and cotton wool. If stippling is produced at the chairside in this way the technician should be warned that after processing the denture this area must be polished with extreme care. A small bristle brush followed by a mop, both mounted in a handpiece, is the method of choice in order to avoid destroying the surface anatomy. A high gloss finish is unnecessary.

An alternative means of applying a stipple finish is by means of the blow-wax technique. A small amount of wax is melted on a spatula and blown onto the wax surface as a spray. The technique is not to be recommended. Not only is the affected surface of variable extent but if carried out at the chairside it will cause the patient to doubt the quality of the operator's cross-infection control practices.

Added realism can be provided by exposing more of the cervical margin of the teeth to stimulate recession, but the illusion has to be maintained by reducing the level of the associated interproximal papillae to give a rounder more flattened tip. At the gingival margin the wax is thickened to imitate a rolled edge. The shape of the gingival crevice can then be reproduced by passing a probe around the gingival margin, the point of the probe being angled at about 20° to the axis of the tooth.

Finally, a word of caution. While precise reproduction of the alveolar and gingival anatomy will please all painstaking clincians it cannot be guaranteed to please all patients. When stippling is present it feels rough to the patient and if the gingivae are reproduced in their rounded, receded form, interproximal spaces are created (especially if tapering form teeth have been chosen which have a contact point near to the incisal edge). Both types of surface finish are more difficult to keep clean and older patients may then find them objectionable. Accurate reproduction of dental and gingival anatomy should not be attempted if it is suspected that adaptation by the patient to the new state will be prolonged or if oral hygiene problems can be anticipated.

Speech

At the try-in stage detection of denture faults from changes in speech is fraught with difficulty and the problem will be approached again in Chapter 8, at which stage diagnosis is easier. Patients adapt rapidly to small changes in tooth site and the majority of phonetic difficulties disappear with time. Only a relatively small number of marked speech faults merit modification of tooth site at this stage if the dentures appear otherwise correct. Because some speech faults are a consequence of poor retention of the bases, before any decisions are made the bases have to be stabilized, if necessary by means of a denture adhesive.

The commoner difficulties are with the labio-dental sounds (the "f" and "v" sounds) when the lower lip is brought into contact with the maxillary anterior teeth. The patient will complain that it is more of an effort to make satisfactory contact if the teeth are further anterior or posterior than previously, and sounds are distorted. Changes in the level of the occlusal plane have the same effect, and if the occlusal plane is higher than the

patient is used to the "v" sound will be converted to a "f". Small changes can be made at this stage to bring the teeth into a more comfortable position but major changes should be avoided unless there is a definite indication on other grounds.

Linguo-dental sounds can be affected by changes in tooth position and the "th" sound will be temporarily different if the maxillary anterior teeth are in a different position to that of the previous denture. Treatment is as for labio-dental difficulties and the patient reassured that adaptation will quickly take place when the permanent prosthesis is made.

Difficulty with "s" and "z" sounds is a more serious fault. If these sounds are converted into a hiss then the face height might be incorrect and the freeway space may have been obliterated. If detected at this stage there is time for a re-try to be made at a reduced face height.

Similarly, difficulties which "ch", "sh" and "j" sounds point to there being an alteration in the space between the arches of the teeth posteriorly with the tongue space being either enlarged or dimished. Theoretically, conversion of the sounds to a hiss should indicate excess space. If the previous denture is available it can be compared with the try-in and the difference in tongue space confirmed. The necessary changes can be made by the technician.

Post dam

Conventionally, the purpose of the post dam, or posterior palatal seal, is to ensure that the saliva film is as thin as possible at the posterior edge of the maxillary denture so that retention is maximized. The post dam should therefore be a zone at the distal edge, where the soft tissues are compressed. The ideal site has been a matter of debate. All agree that the line of compressed tissue should pass through the hamular notches but authorities vary as to the site of the intermediate part and can achieve good retention when placing the post dam at either of the two defined sites. Some advise that it be placed over the hard palate at a point where the underlying bone has sufficient soft tissue over it to allow compression without pressure ulceration of the mucosa. Others advise that the line of the post dam should be sited at the vibrating line which marks the junction between the mobile and immobile areas of the functioning soft palate. Only recently has it been shown by an ultra-sound investigation that the two sites rarely coincide, and that the vibrating line is approximately 3 mm distal to the bony margin of the hard palate in the midline.[2] The investigation also confirmed that a certain amount of latitude exists in the determination of the most effective post dam site.

When making an arbitrary post dam the proposed site on the palate has to be identified. This can be done by palpation of the palate with a ball-ended instrument to identify the compressible site, marking it (the red component of zinc oxide paste is useful) and, if the try-in extends sufficiently far, using it to transfer the mark to the model. Alternatively, the vibrating line can be identified by sight as the patient makes a repeated "ah" sound, marked and transferred in the same way. A simpler method than either is to identify the site of the palatal foveae on either side of the midline near the junction of hard and soft palate. If visible on the model the site for the post dam is marked just in front; if not visible on the model they are identified in the mouth, marked and transferred as before.

In the simplest technique for adjusting the model, the post dam is cut first as an incision with a scalpel into the plaster from one hamular notch to the other through the marked junction, making the incision 1 mm deep at the hamular notches and midline and deeper where there is more soft tissue support. Using the chisel end of a spatula or similar instrument, the anterior margin of the incision is bevelled into a bow shape, taking the convexities of the bow further anteriorly where the initial incision is deeper. After processing, the palatal margin is reduced to a near knife-edge by reduction from the lingual surface. The advantage of the bevel is that if the post dam causes overcompression and pain it can be reduced in depth by cutting it slightly back postero-anteriorly.

A more rational approach to the technique of making a post dam is to analyse the process of denture manufacture and find the real reason for its presence. After packing a flask the acrylic dough is heated to bring about polymerization and arising from the polymerization, volumetric shrinkage of the resin takes place. The shrinkage is not uniform but takes place first in those places where the exotherm of reaction raises the temperature and initiates a more rapid reaction, namely the thicker parts of the base over the crest of the alveolus. Contraction of the dough takes place towards the sites of initial polymerization and because the shape of the space containing the dough provides a physical constraint, a space is created between the polymerizing dough and the palate of the model.[3] In the midline the gap is about 0.5 mm wide, tapering as it passes laterally. On this basis it has been suggested that to compensate for the shrinkage and re-establish contact between the denture and palate, the model should be relieved at the junction of hard and soft palate by cutting a groove with a number 6 round bur. Polymerization shrinkage of this type can also cause tooth movement and account for the occlusal irregularities that can mar the most careful technical work. Such changes are likely to occur in all non-injection moulded work.

Although a variety of techniques have been described for the production of arbitrary post dams involving variable depths of relief and varying degrees of bevelling,[4] all work to the extent that they fill in the gap caused by polymerization shrinkage and in addition thin the saliva film in the post dam region by causing tissue compression. Their complexity is difficulty to justify without being able to calculate accurately the total addition required. Until it can be precisely accounted for, it is probably best to apply a functional post dam at the denture delivery stage.

Additional technical instructions

The additional instructions at this stage may concern the need for minor occlusal adjustments, stippling of the wax surface, the type of resin, and the need for a form of denture identification. At one time, foiling of the working models prior to processing the denture was a common request and was provided not only to make dentures easier to remove from the flask, but to reduce the risk of contamination and discolouration of the denture-base resin by water from the plaster investment. Today this function is provided by an alginate separating medium

and foiling is unnecessary. Foiling of the upper model over the midline raphe or over any palatal torus was also once recommended. It is difficult to justify the process of providing an arbitrary relief in this way when much more precise relief can be given after using disclosing or similar waxes at the chairside once the denture has been inserted.

Foiling of the entire fitting surface of the maxillary model can be justified if the patient suffers from denture stomatitis. The surface that results is easy to keep clean and helps maintain the good oral hygiene so necessary to the permanent control of this annoying condition. The alternative of mechanically polishing the fitting surface is destructive of the base and cannot be advised.

References

1. Lamb, D.J. The effect of Karaya gum on dental enamel. *Br Dent J* **149**:79–82, 1981.
2. Narvekar, R.M. An investigation of the anatomic position of the posterior palatal seal by ultrasound. *J Prosthet Dent* **61**:331–336, 1989.
3. McCartney, J.W. Flange adaptation discrepancy, palatal base distortion and induced malocclusion caused by processing acrylic resin maxillary complete dentures. *J Prosthet Dent* **52**:545–553, 1986.
4. Avant, W.E. A comparison of the retention of complete denture bases having different types of posterior palatal seal. *J Prosthet Dent* **29**:483–493, 1973.

Chapter 6

Denture Processing

Any clinician fully aware of the range of problems which can occur during the processing stages would not relinquish the try-in to his technician lightly and often with so few instructions. Nor would he sleep so easily that night. We have to accept that part of the reason why so many complete dentures are successful and function efficiently lies in the powers of adaptation of our patients. We should acknowledge also that it is due in no small way to the skill of our technicians. The processing of dentures is a job which cannot be allocated to robots, and occasional errors occur as a result of human fallibility. A surprising finding is that mistakes are so rare!

To give the best possible result, close co-operation between the technician and clinician is essential. Despite the sophistication of materials and methods for making denture bases, several problems have yet to be fully overcome, and suggest the ways in which future developments in dental technology may take place. When processing a denture the technician must take care to prevent porosity and dimensional change occurring during the cure and ensure minimal amounts of residual monomer. If it is thought that the base will be inadequately strong then at the clinician's request any necessary reinforcement of the denture base has to be provided.

Problems of denture fracture and tooth loss have to be avoided by ensuring adequate adhesion between the teeth and the base, and special techniques may be prescribed for enhancement of appearance. The decision also has to be made at this stage whether to incorporate some form of patient identification mark in the base and once the denture has been polished it must be disinfected and stored in an appropriate way.

Problems with cure

At present there are three popular heating cycles for the polymerization of heat-cured acrylic resins: a short cure in which the flask is immediately heated up to 100°C by immersion in boiling water, a slow cure in which heating takes place to 72°C and the temperature maintained for 12 or more hours, and an intermediate cycle in which after a period at 72°C, during which polymerization starts, the temperature is raised to 100°C to complete the cure. Choice of cycle can significantly affect the resin properties and determine the type of problem which might arise.

Porosity

Two distinct types of porosity are thought to occur in conventional resins—gaseous and contraction—and are amply described in textbooks. Porosity is said to be common but when present to only a minor degree may be missed, and come to light only when the denture is polished and a layer of porosity encountered below the surface. While it is tempting to repair visible porosity with autopolymerizing resins and so eliminate obvious surface imperfections, the danger always exists that undetected porosity still remains in subsurface layers and can act as a centre for crack initiation. Denture fracture can then follow the application of otherwise sub-critical stresses. Any denture in which porosity is detected should be viewed with suspicion. While it may sometimes be necessary to allow patients to wear porous dentures temporarily—and give a warning that unexpected failure is a possibility—it is best to start replacing the entire denture immediately.

Gaseous porosity is caused by overheating of the resin dough. During the initial phase of curing the exotherm of the polymerization reaction allows localized temperatures higher than those in the surrounding environment. Methyl methacrylate monomer boils at 100.3°C and if the curing temperature is not controlled the boiling point of monomer can be exceeded and porosity follow. Classically, the appearance is of small spherical voids in the centre of the denture-base, or at that part nearer the centre of the flask where the temperature reaches its highest levels. This type of porosity is so well described in textbooks, and so foolproof are the timing mechanisms of the water baths in which dentures are processed that, unless produced deliberately by selecting a short, high-temperature cure, examples should be rare.

Contraction porosity results from excess monomer in the resin dough. Normally the polymer/monomer ratio is between 3.0/1 and 3.5/1 (w/v), at which proportions packing of the dough under pressure compensates for the 7% volumetric shrinkage (approximately 2% linear) that occurs when monomer polymerizes to polymer. When the standard proportion of monomer is exceeded, the polymerization contraction of the mixture may be greater than can be compensated for by compression of the mould and porosity follows. The site and form of contraction porosity are said to differ from that of gaseous porosity, the voids either being irregular and occurring throughout the resin or appearing as surface depressions. The reason for this is that polymerization first takes place centrally, where the temperatures are higher, and compensation for shrinkage of the excess monomer is provided for by contraction of more peripheral areas. Later when the more peripheral areas polymerize, gross uncompensated shrinkage results, and surface depressions or voids within the mass of the dough are formed as uncured material is drawn towards the centres of polymerization. Contraction porosity may be distributed generally throughout the denture base, or can be localized. The latter phenomenon is a result of localized excess of monomer arising from inadequate mixing.

The above explanations are intellectually satisfying and provide a physicochemical basis for the extreme types of porosity. However, while gaseous and contraction porosity may both be rationally explained and their characteristic appearances defined, recent research has shown that the situation in real life is far from simple.[1] While porosity can apparently be induced under three very different conditions, namely by mixing dough with excess monomer, underpacking, or heating excessively, the resulting forms of porosity are classical in neither shape nor distribution. All that can be confirmed is that thin sections are more likely to be free of voids than thick sections, which emphasizes the relative importance of the increase in temperature caused by the exotherm. Whether the resulting porosity is due to vapourization of the monomer or its contraction on polymerization must remain a source of debate. Even the possibility that porosity is in part caused by the inclusion of air cannot be eliminated.

If we assume that the dough has not been overmixed to the extent that air has been incorporated, then a plausible explanation may be that both gaseous and contraction porosity tend to occur simultaneously. If, to avoid air being incorporated, mixing is minimal, it is likely that there are sites where excess monomer is present. The polymerization exotherm can then produce high temperatures locally and a hot-spot results with the production of mixed porosity, partly due to overheating and partly due to uncompensated contraction. To avoid porosity every effort must be made to eliminate excess monomer by strict adherence to the advised proportions of powder and liquid.

A third form of porosity is granular porosity, which results from a lack of monomer, and consequently insufficient matrix to completely surround the polymer particles. This can result when the dough has been left unused, and exposed to air, for a prolonged period of time. Surface momomer then has time to evaporate and after processing, a characteristic opaque, streaky surface results.

Residual monomer

Even after careful processing of a conventional pack and press heat-cured acrylic denture-base resin there may remain a proportion of residual monomer, the amount varying between 0.2% and 0.4%.[2] Several defects are attributed to its presence. Its plasticizing effect will reduce the mechanical strength of the base and by allowing stress relief can cause dimensional change following removal of the denture from the model. At concentrations over 1.0% it can cause a mucosal reaction in sensitive patients.

The major factors involved in ensuring that residual monomer levels in heat-cured resins are as low as possible appear to be the temperature and time of cure. For the sake of speed, short curing cycles have been devised, with immediate curing temperatures of 100°C which are maintained for only short periods of time. Such methods have been shown to result in levels of residual monomer 3–4 times higher than those which involve cure at low temperatures for prolonged periods (72°C for about 12 hours).[3] With proper anticipation of working practices the extra curing time required for more complete polymerization is unlikely to affect the total technical time, and hence the cost, unless speed is at a high premium.

Dimensional changes

During the process of making a denture from a conventional resin, dimensional changes occur. These may be a consequence of poor technique when packing the resin dough or they may occur during curing of the base. Even after processing and removal of the denture from the model some dimensional changes occur following water sorption and stress relief.

When dimensional changes occur during packing, the cause is technical error as a consequence of damaging pressure exerted on the teeth during flask closure. If the dough is too stiff the pressure needed to close the flask can cause one or more teeth to be forced into the plaster. Alternatively, if the plaster is weak due to excess water, or the inclusion or air bubbles, even normal pressures are sufficient to cause crushing of the plaster. The inevitable result of either mishap will be a prominent tooth or cusp.

A relative movement of all teeth may occur if excess flash remains on closure of the flask. Rarely, this may be the result of inadequate pressure being applied when closing the flask. More likely, it will be due to use of an excessively stiff dough, itself caused by too low a powder/liquid ratio or too much time elapsing after initial mixing, so allowing the dough to stiffen beyond its working consistency.

Significant defects can also occur during processing, with measurable distortion of the denture-base. The principal source of error is polymerization contraction, which has been shown to cause changes in the position of the teeth and to the fitting surfaces of the denture.[4] Most importantly for the clinician, contact is lost between the fitting surface of the palate and the underlying soft tissues. As with the case for levels of residual monomer, the changes have been found to be greatest when a short, high-temperature cure was used.

Even after prescribing a long, low-temperature cure some dimensional changes occur. Techniques and materials have therefore been devised for reducing the clinical effect of dimensional changes.

Split cast technique

Because unwanted tooth movements are common and may be said to be inevitable, the technique of split cast mounting has been developed which allows minor occlusal errors to be corrected before the dentures are inserted. In this technique the working models have their bases scored and a separating agent applied before being mounted on the articulator by means of the occlusal rec-

ord made at the registration stage. Following a successful try-in, the working models are removed from the plaster attaching them to the mounting bases on the arms of the articulator. After again coating with separating medium (a solution of detergent is adequate) the working models and try-in are invested and the denture processed as normal.

The flask is carefully separated after processing and the investing plaster removed from the working model and its attached denture. The working models are now replaced on the articulator bases, sealed with sticky wax or contact adhesive and the occlusal surfaces re-adjusted into balanced articulation, first into the intercuspal position and then into lateral excursions. The technique is excellent for eliminating premature contacts caused by movement of individual teeth or small numbers of teeth. Provided that the increase in face height has not been too great it can also be used to correct increases in face height caused by excess flash. The technique should not be used as an alternative to careful technical procedures and it cannot compensate for any changes caused by stress relaxation or water sorption following removal of the denture from the model. It works best when every effort is made to ensure dimensional stability.

Pour resins

Because changes in occlusal relations are common when using conventional heat-cured resins, techniques of producing dentures by means of autopolymerizing, or cold-cure, resins have been promoted. These have the advantage that the process of denture manufacture does not involve a flask with two separate parts and usually the only pressure applied to the setting resin is that resulting from placing it in a pressurized container.

Consequently, there is no flash to cause an increase in face height, and movement of teeth into the investing material under the influence of unidirectional pressure is unlikely.

Unfortunately there are unwanted side effects. Porosity is not unusual in dentures made with "pour" type resins, and tends to occur in those parts of the denture which are uppermost in the mould, especially if the resin is allowed to stiffen beyond a point of maximum fluidity. While the processing stages are easier and cleaner, pour resins have a low powder/liquid ratio and during polymerization the large amount of monomer contracts to an extent which it may be impossible to compensate for. Although the proponents of pour resins emphasize the smaller amount of technical work needed to produce a denture by this means, the technique requires considerably more care for a faultless result and more time may be needed after processing to repair porosity. The molecular weight of autopolymerizing resins is less than conventional heat-cured resins and has in the past led to their criticism on the grounds of inferior mechanical strength and lack of fracture resistance. Nevertheless, the physical properties of the pour resins have been much improved of late and a recently described modification which involves curing first under vacuum and then under pressure gives an acrylic resin with properties comparable with conventional denture resins.[5] Unfortunately, the presence of large amounts of residual monomer may still cause sensitivity in susceptible subjects.

The technique of making dentures with pour resins first involves trimming the axial surfaces of the working models to a slightly conical shape. After placing model and try-in on the base of a duplicating flask or similar container, they are invested in reversible hydrocolloid. After

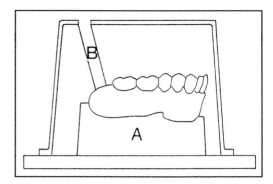

Fig. 6.1 Cross-section showing technique of denture manufacture with "pour" resin. A, tapered model. B, access channel for resin.

it has set, the model and try-in are removed (easily done if the axial surfaces of the model have been correctly trimmed) and access channels bored, through the investment, connecting the surface to unimportant but accessible parts of the future denture—usually the retromolar region of mandibular dentures or the tuberosity region of maxillary dentures (Fig. 6.1).

After removing the try-in from the model the denture teeth and the working model are replaced and a fluid mix of resin poured down one access channel, taking care to avoid air inclusions. Cure take place under pressure in a hydroflask at a slightly increased temperature (about 45°C), but not so high that the hydrocolloid investment liquefies. The resulting surface detail of the denture is excellent and little finishing and polishing are required unless porosity is present. The finances of the process are complex. While technical time is saved by the simplified processing, the materials are costly and repair of visible porosity is a possible extra expense. Investigations of the subject have shown that few savings are made unless the time factor is of great importance.[6]

Injection moulding

An alternative means of improving the accuracy of denture-base processing is by injection moulding which eliminates errors due to the presence of a flash. The original methods involved injecting a fluid thermoplastic resin (polymethyl methacrylate, Nylon and polycarbonate can be used) into a mould under high pressure and temperature. An accurate, highly cross-linked denture base could be made but the expense was considerable and today may only be justified if a patient is either allergic to acrylic or requires a fatigue-resistant base. The two needs could be met by a denture-base made of polycarbonate.

Denture fracture and reinforcement

Fracture of dentures is common, the total NHS cost for denture repairs in the UK being in excess of £5 million annually. While the bulk strength properties of poly (methyl methacrylate) are sufficient for most purposes, a denture will break if the thickness of resin is insufficient for the stresses imposed on it. Fracture is therefore especially common when the interalveolar space is restricted due to large residual ridges or when a denture is made for a patient with a powerfully developed masticatory musculature. When a denture-base has fractured completely, it is usually repaired as quickly as possible but small discrepancies in localization of the pieces ensure that both the fitting and occlusal surfaces are an imprecise fit. Although the strength of a repair can be near that of intact resins, the mismatch between the occlusal and fitting surfaces concentrates stresses at the joint and will cause another fracture unless at a later visit the repaired denture

is relined and the occlusal surface re-adjusted into balance.

Diagnosis

A fracture during function usually initiates from a surface crack, defect, or area of stress concentration, hence the importance of ensuring a porosity-free resin. Anatomical factors may be responsible by producing an initial surface notch or defect. Such factors include fraenal notches (especially the maxillary labial fraenum which is often well developed), and bony, prominences. Fracture can also occur due to fatigue following continual flexing of a maxillary denture, during mastication, over a prominent midline torus. More recently, the importance has been stressed of sites where the surface of the resin is indented by the presence of porcelain teeth or by acrylic teeth which have not achieved an adequate chemical bond. An SEM study has shown that signs typical of crack initiation can be detected where incompletely bonded teeth cause a defect of the surface integrity.[7]

When a patient has broken a denture it is important to first identify the cause of fracture before attempting repair or replacement. The denture may have broken after impact—typically after being dropped. In many cases this is pure accident and little can be done apart from repairing it. Often fracture occurs while the dentures are being cleaned and many such accidents can be prevented by warning patients at the stage of denture delivery to take care and ensure that a bowl of water, towel, or suitable soft surface is put beneath the site of operation. When the cause of the accident is the patient's unsteadiness—and many of our patients are elderly—then replacement of the denture by one made from a high-impact acrylic may be the solution.

The cause of the fracture is often a mechanical defect and examination of the fracture surface will reveal signs of porosity, contamination by a foreign body or previous repair. Crack propagation can start from such a defect and will progress gradually until the denture fractures in the course of normal mastication. Although the denture may then be repaired as a temporary measure, a new denture should be made as soon as possible. Provided it is made with care, conventional resin will be adequately strong.

Alternatively, examination of the mouth may reveal a large fraenum, prominent torus or inadequate interalveolar space. While a new denture can be made, it too will fracture unless the anatomical problem is first removed. If this is impossible for reasons of health or because the patient refuses surgical treatment, then a cast metal base must be provided.

Methods of denture base reinforcement

Mechanical reinforcement of an acrylic denture-base may be either by inclusions or by prefabricating a metal base. Both have their advantages and disadvantages.

Reinforcement by inclusions

If a patient gives a history of having dropped a denture and it is suspected that this will be a common future occurrence, a high impact resin may be the material of choice for the replacement. High-impact acrylic is a co-polymer of acrylic and butadiene (the polymer part is a mixture of acrylic and rubber particles) and forms a matrix of acrylic with inclusions of rubber. In this way crack propagation is inhibited, the rubber inclusions serving to prevent crack progress. Although the material will resist impact

fracture,[8] it is no stronger—rather less strong—than a conventional resin,[9] and high impact resins should not be used if the cause of fracture is a mechanical or anatomical fault.

For many years attempts have been made to improve the strength of acrylic resin by incorporating strengthening materials. The first of these were meshes of various metals. Although the meshes themselves were strong and prevented separation of the parts of the denture when fracture had occurred, fracture of the resin was not prevented, indeed the remaining resin was weaker on account of its diminished bulk. Alternative reinforcing agents have included fibres of various types. Such reinforcement is at its most efficient when the fibres can be orientated at right angles to the likely line of fracture. Unfortunately, when using current methods of base manufacture, techniques involving the use of oriented fibres are possible only with the expenditure of additional time and expense, although greatly increased fatigue strength is shown by acrylic resin reinforced with mats of glass fibre or carbon fibre.[10]

In order to allow cheapness of manufacture compatible with near-normal techniques, fibres have been introduced with random orientation, most often glass fibre, carbon fibre, ultra-high modulus polyethylene, or aramid (Kevlar) fibre. Despite some improvements in strength, results have been disappointing. On physical grounds this has been in part due to the low proportion of fibre that can be intoduced without affecting the handling properties of the dough and in part because only a proportion of the fibre is orientated in a direction which allows maximum resistance to applied forces. Primarily, it has been because in the absence of a suitable agent to bond the included fibre to the acrylic matrix it is difficult to achieve the improvements in strength which can be expected in similar industrial applications where bonding is possible.[11] On clinical grounds there have been further complications, in part due to the unacceptable colour of some fibres (carbon fibre is black), and in part due to mucosal irritation encountered when a stiff fibre is exposed into the mouth on polishing the resin base.

Reinforcement with metal bases

To date, developments in composite-type denture-base resins have not achieved the dramatic results seen in the field of composite resins for conservative dentistry. Where great strength in thin section is important or resistance to fatigue fracture is considered essential, then the only satisfactory reinforcement for an acrylic denture is a metal base. Stainless steel has the advantage of being thinner and tougher, but its mode of manufacture (by hydraulic pressing on a specially strengthened die) makes it expensive. This, in association with the extreme difficulty encountered in making any necessary adjustments to a stainless steel base and the need for welded tagging to ensure mechanical attachment of the resin base, have popularized the use of cast metals.

Most such bases are made of cobalt/chromium alloys which have their own, but lesser, problems. When used to strengthen a mandibular denture the ridge is normally well formed and to allow the anterior teeth to be sited in a restricted space without contacting the base, it is normally designed to cover only the lingual surface of the ridge anteriorly and terminate at the crest, so leaving the labial surface free. The maxillary metal base is similar in design and covers the palate to the crest of the ridge (where mechanical attachment for the acrylic is incorporated) and back to the post dam region. A difficulty sometimes encountered with the maxillary denture is that of adding a functional post dam when retention proves to be inadequate. Adhesion of added acrylic to the metal base is normally poor, but a technique has been described for attaching acrylic to cobalt/chromium alloy by first acid-etching to secure good micromechanical locking.[12]

The most recent development in adhesive technology has been the introduction of an acrylic resin which is adhesive to metal. By incorporating 5% 4 META (4-methacryloxyethyl trimellitate anhydride) in the monomer, the adhesive bond is greatly improved.[13] While the implications for orthodontics and partial denture prosthodontics are significant, even in complete denture prosthodontics the design of metal bases can be simplified with a reduction in cost.

Bonding between tooth and base

The two materials available for the manufacture of denture teeth—procelain and acrylic—have differing mechanisms for attachment to the denture base. The attachment of porcelain teeth is by means of gold plated pins or diatoric holes. Retention of porcelain teeth is normally excellent, although loss occasionally occurs following corrosion of the pins, or when there is reduced interalveolar space and much of the diatoric hole has been removed in order to fit the tooth into the limited available space.

Loss of acrylic teeth is more common, despite being able to achieve a chemical bond with the denture base. When acrylic teeth are lost it can be presumed that the adhesive bond between the tooth and the base is inadequate. For a satisfactory chemical bond absolute cleanliness of the denture tooth is vital, and contamination with inadequately boiled out wax appears to be the major problem,[14] although contact of teeth with misdirected cold mould seal has to be scrupulously avoided. In order to improve the area of contact between the tooth and the resin base the fitting surface of the tooth can be roughened with a stone prior to packing the dough. This has the additional advantage of removing any remaining adherent surface contaminants.

Wiping the fitting surface of denture teeth with methyl methacrylate monomer has also been suggested as a means of improving the adhesive bond by softening the tooth surface. In many cases the rationale for this is unsound. While monomer will soften non-cross-linked resins, the majority of cheaper denture teeth are made entirely of highly cross-linked resin and are not soluble. Unless the manufacturers have constructed the denture teeth in resin layers of varying degrees of cross-linking (which is the case with some of the more expensive varieties) the action is of limited value. Without contacting the suppliers to confirm the method of manufacture, wiping with mono(methyl methacrylate) serves little purpose beyond aiding the cleansing of the tooth surface.

Newer processing methods

While the traditional ways of curing denture base resins give satisfactory results, research is constantly taking place to improve the accuracy of the finished product and make the process more convenient. The latest methods include modified injection moulding, microwave curing and light curing.

Modified injection moulding

A less costly variation of injection moulding is now available which in-

volves injection of a conventional resin dough under high pressure. The reasoning is that this method compensates for polymerization shrinkage by forcing extra resin into the flask. Because flask closure takes place before pressure injection of resin starts, no flash is produced and occlusal faults are reduced in frequency. The modified form of injection moulding, while more expensive than conventional dough and press methods, is less so than the original type of injection moulding, and is the processing method recommended by one large manufacturer of prosthetic materials (Ivoclar, Leichtenstein). Although the technique gave excellent results in trials on non-anatomic dies,[15] it still does not eliminate errors occurring during the clinical stages and cannot act as a substitute for a final check record.

Microwave curing

Conventional microwave ovens generate a microwave of frequency 2450 MHz which acts to increase directly the energy levels of water molecules. A new development has been the adaptation of the principle to curing of acrylic resin doughs, the microwave frequency produced by a conventional microwave oven also serving to energize the acrylic monomer molecule. Rapid cure takes place, but with some uneven heating unless a mechanism is incorporated to rotate the flask or otherwise alter its position within the microwave beam. The technique is in its infancy at present and the results, while excellent on the grounds of producing a distortion-free base, cannot compare with conventional methods on the grounds of expense. Complex electronic equipment is required and unless the generator is tuned to a shorter wavelength, special non-metallic fibre-reinforced flasks are needed to provent arcing.[16] In time, capital equipment costs will fall if the technique becomes popular. In years to come microwave curing may provide a method of denture-base production for those cases where a high-quality, speedy result is essential. At present it is principally a research toy, but microwave ovens can be used more conventionally for the making of facial prostheses when they help to dry out and strengthen the unwieldy models.[16]

Light-cured denture base resins

Development of light-cured composite resins was quickly followed by a light-cured denture base resin, the resin being provided in the form of dough-like, partly polymerized, sheets, ropes and blocks. The process is well established for the manufacture of orthodontic appliances but its application to complete denture prosthodontics is complicated because of the need to provide access for the activating light. Its clinical applications are likely to be in the field of additions and relines, but special trays can be made (rather expensively) by this method. Appliances produced by this method show excellent dimensional stability, good mechanical properties, and low residual monomer but have the disadvantage that there is a certain amount of porosity and, because water sorption is of the order of 3–4%, the end product is liable to stain.[18]

Denture identification

Ideally all dentures should have an identification mark in the unlikely event that it is required for forensic purposes. A more common situation is when the dentures of patients in hospitals or nursing homes are mislaid, and then the presence of a name is invaluable. Three methods are available for identification of dentures. The first can be applied at the packing stage and involves including an identification label in the denture flask. Some time and effort has to be put into making the labels beforehand, but the method gives a permanent result. However, despite being permanent, most such methods can be criticized on the grounds that it is difficult to prevent movement of the label during the packing of the flask and it can subsequently be easily displaced or distorted. Further, unless it bonds to acrylic resin it will form a point of weakness and if it comes to the surface when polishing or adjusting, it will cause microleakage and irritation unless recovered with another layer of resin.

The cheapest and most satisfactory method for permanent identification at this stage involves making the label in acrylic resin. A small amount of clear autopolymerizing acrylic is allowed to set between two glass sheets separated by a 0.25 mm spacer made of orthodontic ligature wire. One side is roughened by sandblasting and then the sheet is scored and broken into strips 5 mm wide. The patient's details—normally the first six letters of their name plus their postal code—are written in reverse on the sandblasted side of a short strip using a fine fibre-tipped pen. After performing a trial closure the flask is opened and the strips placed marked surface down on the fitting surface of the dough. Only if the label is made of acrylic will it bond with the denture base and not act as a source of weakness and only if it is very thin will the pressure of flask closure adapt it closely to the surface of the working model. The thickness of the label separates the lettering from the surface and prevents it being removed by normal denture cleansing methods (Fig. 6.2). By inserting the label after trial closure little further dough movement takes place and even if a moderate amount occurs the

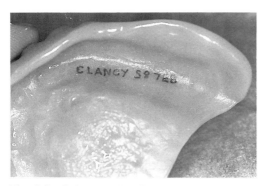

Fig. 6.2 A denture identified by incorporation an acrylic label prior to processing.

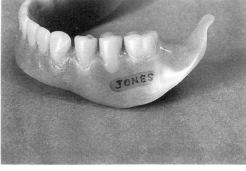

Fig. 6.3 Denture marked by cutting a channel and writing the patient's name with a fibre-tipped pen. The channel is filled with autopolymerizing resin.

label is restrained by its contact with the model surface.

The second method involves cutting a relief chamber in the finished denture, 1 mm or more deep, and large enough either to allow the details to be written on the base with a spirit-based fibre-tip pen, or for a label to be introduced. The relief chamber is then filled with clear cold-cure acrylic and re-polished (Fig. 6.3). This method requires a little extra time and a certain amount of special equipment but is permanent and problem-free once it has been applied. Those who have described the method[19] warn of the dangers of porosity when an incompatible label is inserted, or reaction between monomer and some marking inks, and of slight loss of visibility with time.

The third method can be used when circumstances arise which warrant it, and is applied to dentures in use. It involves placing names or codes on the intact surface of the denture and protecting the letters with a surface film. It will be dealt with in Chapter 7.

None of the above methods should be used without a little diplomatic explanation. While the majority of patients accept denture identificaton without demur, some insist on it being placed on

the fitting surface where it is least likely to be seen. A few refuse outright. Of these some are averse to the idea of being labelled, and others dislike the intimations of mortality involved in a forensic marking system.

The amount of information to put in an identification mark can be debated. For forensic purposes the post code is sufficient, but for patients in hospital or nursing home whose memories may be untrustworthy, the name is essential. A compromise is a combination of initials and post code with the addition of the year of manufacture if the clinician feels that a review reminder is needed.

Colour modification of denture bases

The appearance of denture base materials is excellent. The general colour is achieved by ball-milling pigments into the acrylic beads, and red Nylon filaments can be included to add the appearance of small blood vessels. Manufacturers even market a range of acrylics in which the normal pink pigment has had blue and black modifiers added to imitate the melanin pigmented gingival tissues found in many patients and especially in those of non-Caucasian races. Modified acrylics are used in exactly the same way as normal acrylics.

With a little extra work it is possible, when using conventionally cured denture-bases, to imitate the variation in shade that the natural gingivae show. One way is to incorporate coloured Nylon strands which imitate local deposits of melanin. Additions are made at the dough stage but due to movements of the dough during packing it is difficult to provide other than a random distribution. A better way is to use a denture stain kit, consisting of a range of pigmented acrylic polymers which are added to the dough before final processing.

Two techniques are popular for adding pigmented acrylics. In one they are added in thin layers to the surfaces of the investment plaster after the wax try-in has been boiled out and the investing plaster has been dried. Taking care not to disturb the teeth, red stained acrylic is added in the region of the attached gingivae and pale pink over the alveolar prominences. The "drop" technique is used for building up the layers, acrylic being added after dipping the tip of a fine brush moistened with monomer into the polymer beads and transferring the resulting bead to the position required. Layers of added acrylic are thinned at the periphery where it has to blend in with normal acrylic. Once all layers of acrylic have been added the flask is packed and processed normally, but with care to avoid damage to the pigmented layers.

An alternative method allows a better idea of the final result before processing. The wax try-in is boiled out and the flask packed with dough as normal, but a trial closure made with a sheet of polythene film between the teeth and the dough, rather than between the dough and the model. After separating the halves of the flask, pigmented acrylic is added directly to the dough to achieve the effect required. Subsequently the final closure is made and processing follows as normal. With either technique care has to be taken during finishing or the thin pigmented layers will be removed by overzealous polishing.

Storage

A recent study has shown that the majority of dentures returned from laboratories are contaminated, sometimes with pathogenic organisms.[20] With the current emphasis on cross-infection control measures it is important that the finished denture cannot be suspected of being infected. When technical procedures are complete the denture is disinfected in a solution of 1% glutaraldehyde for 15 minutes before being washed and placed in a sealed container of sterile water. Storage in water is preferred to storage under dry conditions in order to allow water sorption to take place. Although the reasons for this action are theoretically sound and allow any expansion and stress relaxation to take place, despite up to 2% water uptake by weight, the dimensional changes, at less than 1%, are probably clinically insignificant.

References

1. Wolfaardt, J.F., Cleaton-Jones, P. and Fatti, P. The occurance of porosity in a heat-cured poly (methyl methacrylate) denture base resin. *J Prosthet Dent* **55**:393–400, 1986.
2. Austin, A.T. and Basker, R.M. The level of residual monomer in acrylic denture base materials. *Br Dent J* **149**:281–286, 1980.
3. Honorez, P., Catalan, A., Angnes, U. and

Grimonster, J. The effect of three processing cycles on some physical and chemical properties of a heat-cured acrylic resin. *J Prosthet Dent* **61**:510–517, 1989.

4. McCartney, J.W. Flange adaptation discrepancy, palatal base distortion and induced malocclusion caused by processing acrylic resin maxillary complete dentures. *J Prosthet Dent* **52**:545–553, 1984.

5. Frangou, M., Huggett, R. and Stafford, G.D. Evaluation of the properties of a new pour denture base material utilising a modified technique and initiator system. *J Oral Rehabil* **17**:67–77, 1990.

6. Bates, J.F., Stafford, G.D., Huggett, R. and Handley, R.W. Current status of pour type denture base resins. *J Dent* **5**:177–189, 1977.

7. Lamb, D.J., Ellis, B. and van Noort, R. The fracture topography of acrylic dentures broken in service. *Biomaterials* **6**:110–112, 1985.

8. Neihart, T.R. and Flinton, R.J. Measuring fracture toughness of high-impact poly (methyl methacrylate) with the short rod method. *J Prosthet Dent* **60**:249–253, 1988.

9. Chitchumnong, P., Brooks, S.C. and Stafford, G.D. Comparison of three- and four-point flexural strength of denture base polymers. *Dent Mater* **5**:2–5, 1989.

10. Bowman, A.J. and Manley, T.R. The elimination of breakages in upper dentures by reinforcement with carbon fibre. *Br Dent J* **156**:87–89,

11. Grave, A.M.H., Chandler, H.D. and Wolfaardt, J.F. Denture base acrylic reinforced with high modulus fibre. *Dent Mater* **1**:185–187, 1985.

12. Garfield, R.E. An effective method for relining metal–based prostheses with acid etch techniques. *J Prosthet Dent* **53**:719–721, 1984.

13. Jacobson, T.E., Chai Chang J., Keri, P.P. and Watanabe, L.G. Bond strength of 4-META acrylic resin denture base to cobalt chromium alloy. *J Prosthet Dent* **60**:570–576, 1988.

14. Spratley, M.H. An investigation of the adhesion of acrylic resin teeth to dentures. *J Prosthet Dent* **58**:389–392, 1987.

15. Anderson, G.C., Schulte, J.K. and Arnold, T.G. Dimensional stability of injection and conventional processing of denture base acrylic. *J Prosthet Dent* **60**:394–398, 1988.

16. De Clerk, J.P. Microwave polymerization of acrylic resins used in dental prosthesis. *J Prosthet Dent* **57**:650–658, 1987.

17. Seals, R.R., Cortes, A.L., Funk, J.J. and Parel, S.M. Microwave technique for fabrication of provisional facial prosthesis. *J Prosthet Dent* **62**:327–331, 1989.

18. Kahn, Z., von Fraunhofer, J.A. and Razavi, R. The staining characteristics, transverse strength and micro-hardness of a visible light-cured denture base material. *J Prosthet Dent* **57**:384–386, 1987.

19. Fletcher, A.M., Turner, C.H. and Ritchie, G.M. Denture marking methods and induced stress. *Br Dent J* **142**:224–226, 1977.

20. Wakefield, C.W. Laboratory contamination of dental prosthesis. *J Prosthet Dent* **44**:143–146, 1980.

Chapter 7

Denture Delivery

A variety of problems can arise at the denture delivery stage, including pain, lack of retention, occlusal defects and nausea. Any one of them can dishearten even the most optimistic of patients. Usually they consider this the most important of their visits and may have been looking forward to it for some time. To preserve confidence it is essential that no patient leaves the surgery with an unsatisfactory denture. All problems of pain, retention or occlusion must be eliminated at this stage which, if necessary, can be prolonged over two visits. If nausea is complained of, it must be treated or at least reassurance given, and finally, before the patient leaves the surgery the need for denture identification should be considered.

The most pressing problem is always pain. For the sake of simplicity, the types of pain may be classified according to the stage at which they are encountered. Pain may occur immediately on insertion of the denture and can be eliminated by adjustment of the fitting surface, or alternatively, the pain may arise on occluding the teeth and require treatment after occlusal adjustment has been performed.

Pain on insertion

Although gross undercuts will have been blocked out on the master model before processing the denture and the technician will have subsequently made every effort to remove visible imperfections from the fitting surface, sources of pain sometimes still remain and require attention. Any remaining undercuts in the denture-base cause pain on insertion as the base shears past the prominence of the undercut alveolus, and the pain is eliminated by adjustment of the fitting surface, not over the site of pain, but peripheral to the depression in the base caused by the alveolar prominence. Care must be taken at the same time to maintain stability by preserving the length of the associated flange. This is especially relevant when removing undercuts related to the mylohyoid ridge both at, and distal to, the insertion to the mylohyoid muscle. If part of the flange extension can be preserved it will provide added stability for the mandibular denture by its interaction with the lateral surface of the tongue (Fig. 7.1A and B).

Pimples of acrylic on the fitting surface of a denture are difficult to see and are the result of penetration of acrylic, under pressure, into small air bubbles beneath the surface of the model. They always cause pain but fortunately patients can usually locate them accurately and direct the operator to their site when they can be palpated and removed.

Once initial causes of pain have been identified and corrected, the removal of

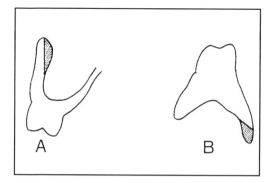

Fig. 7.1 Method of reduction of over-extended denture base. Shaded sections are to be removed. A, undercut in maxillary molar region. B, retromylohyoid region.

further painful pressure points is left until after the elimination of faults of retention and occlusion. Many apparent pressure spots are due to premature occlusal contacts and to avoid confusion it is better to delay further investigation of pain untl later in the visit.

Lack of retention

A frustrated clinician sometimes uses "denture warpage" as an excuse when it proves difficult to rectify a retention problem. Small dimensional changes do occur during processing[1] but can be compensated for. Provided adequate investigation of potential problems has been carried out at the assessment stage, then if the denture still lacks retention at the end of the delivery stage, a defect of the operator's clinical skills is more likely than technical failure.

At this stage lack of retention may have one of a number of primary causes. If a maxillary denture is unretentive at rest or during speech the problem is usually lack of peripheral seal or else underextension, rarely is it overextension. The reason is that if extension and peripheral seal are adequate, retention of a maxillary denture will be so good that overextension of the periphery will cause pain rather than denture displacement. If lack of peripheral seal is suspected the site must be identified. First, the adequacy of the post dam is tested by pressing the maxillary denture firmly into place, then tilting it down at the back. If the denture is easily displaced the lack of retention is rectified by adding a functional post dam with autopolymerizing acrylic.

The procedure is as follows. First, check that the denture has been fully extended to the junction of hard and soft palate and remove the remains of any arbitrary post dam that has already been placed. Mix a small amount of autopolymerizing acrylic resin and, when it has reached a manipulable state, place it as a beading across the posterior edge of the fitting surface from one hamular notch to the other. Wait until the resin has reached a dough-like state, then replace the denture and ask the patient to occlude firmly for a few seconds. Remove it and allow the resin to polymerize rapidly in warm water. Best results are achieved if a pressure flask is available to ensure a non-porous resin and further accelerate the rate of set. Finally, surplus resin that has extruded beyond the limit of the denture is removed and any rough surfaces polished.

In a similar way impression wax can be used to produce a post dam. Melted wax is applied with a brush to the post dam region, immersed in cold water and then the denture placed in the mouth under occlusal pressure for 6 minutes.[2] Further additions are made unless there is visible evidence by dulling of the surface that contact has been made over the entire width of the palate. The seal is then replaced in heat-cured acrylic resin, using a prolonged cure cycle to minimize distortion.

Some operators prefer to place a post dam at the chairside always, rather than rely on arbitrary carving of the working model at the try-in stage. Their rationale has been explained in an earlier chapter and is that the need for a post dam on a maxillary denture follows from a lack of fit over the hard palate, which is caused in turn by polymerization contraction of the denture-base resin during processing.[3] As a consequence of the chemical exotherm, the processing temperature is higher in the thicker parts of the denture over the crest of the ridge and contraction of the dough occurs towards these zones of rapid initial cure. Uncured resin in the palate is pulled towards the zones of initial cure, opening up a gap between the fitting surface of the denture and the model. Carving a post dam at the try-in stage closes the gap in an arbitrary way and a more precise method is to fill it with a functionally developed post dam.

As a corollary, some cases of poorly retentive maxillary dentures result from palatal underextension associated with the cutting of an excessive arbitrary post dam. The central section of the post dam then abuts against relatively incompressible tissue and the close fit necessary for secure retention is lost. In these cases retention can be perceptibly improved by removing the post dam.

When retention of a maxillary denture is still poor despite adequate retention in the post dam region an alternative site for underextension of the periphery must be suspected, and it can usually be detected by holding the denture in place and tilting it from side to side when loss of retention will indicate the site of underextension. To rectify the fault, the periphery is extended by means of a local impression made in zinc oxide/eugenol impression paste, supported if necessary by a preliminary addition of Greenstick composition or a functional trim material based on silicone or autopolymerizing butyl methacrylate resin. The addition can be completed by being replaced in autopolymerizing resin, but with its attendant problems. Ideally such additions should be completed in heat-cured resin, but taking care to maintain the processing temperature at 72°C for a prolonged cure, otherwise stress relief can cause distortion of the denture base.

A functional seal is more difficult to achieve in the complex muscular environment at the periphery of a mandibular denture and here lack of retention is commonly due to extension of the denture over muscle attachments. Diagnosis of a lingual overextension is made by maintaining the denture in position in the mouth with the forefingers and encouraging tongue movements by the patient. Certain specific faults are easily detected. Displacement when the tongue is protruded and the palatoglossus muscle passively drawn forwards indicates overextension in the posterior lingual region where the palatoglossus marks the distal end of the lingual sulcus. Similarly, extension of the base over the attachment of the genioglossus to the superior genial tubercle is diagnosed by displacement of the base when this muscle is stretched by raising and retracting the tongue. Extension over the attachment of the mylohyoid muscle to the mylohyoid ridge is diagnosed by pain when, with the mouth closed, the tongue is pressed against the hard palate and the mylohyoid contracts to raise the floor of the mouth. Alternatively, with the mouth partly open and the denture supported by the fingers, the tongue can be protruded to touch the corners of the mouth alternately. Functional overextension beyond the insertion of the mylohyoid is then revealed when the denture lifts on the side opposite to the tip of the tongue. If it can be tolerated, try to make the reduction from the lingual surface to preserve the extension.

As a cause of lack of retention, buccal overextension is easy to suspect but more difficult to prove. Contrary to popular belief, the buccinator muscle need not be attached solely to the external oblique ridge but can arise anywhere on the buccal shelf between the external oblique ridge laterally and the crest of the residual ridge medially. Further, the degree to which a denture can overlie the insertion without being displaced is variable and is probably determined by the intrinsic level of activity of the patient's facial musculature. If the correct extent of the buccal periphery has been determined at the impression stage by means of a functionally extended impression, the best course of action is to resist any temptation to extend or reduce it at the delivery stage. Instead, leave it to the review stage when any painful overextension can be adjusted in response to the patient's reaction.

In cases where underextension of the mandibular denture-base is suspected, additions to the periphery can be made in the same way as with a maxillary denture. A simpler alternative, when general underextension is suspected, is to reline or rebase the entire denture using a functional trim material to establish the new periphery, followed by a wash of zinc oxide/eugenol or fluid silicone rubber. This procedure will increase the face height slightly and is acceptable only when there is no danger of intruding into the interocclusal space.

Occlusal irregularities

Small defects of the occlusal surface are often discovered when checking tooth contact. While registering the jaw relations, precise location of the blocks is difficult if they are not perfectly stable or if the ridges are very resorbed. Inevitably there will be some defect of the final occlusion. Further, even after the most perfect jaw registration technique, slight tooth displacement can occur during processing if the acrylic dough is stiff and/or the presence of air bubbles renders the plaster investment weak. Many of the smaller occlusal irregularities that are detected can be corrected by adjustment in the mouth at the chairside or, after transfer of the malocclusion to an articulator, by a check record or remount procedure. When the occlusal irregularity is more than slight or includes an antero-posterior or lateral discrepancy a check record is essential.

Chairside technique

Two materials are in common use to aid identification and adjustment of occlusal high spots at the chairside. The most popular and cheapest is articulating paper. After inserting the dentures, and if necessary stabilizing the mandibular denture with denture fixative, a horseshoe of articulating paper—the thinnest types give the best results—is placed over the occlusal surface of the mandibular denture and the patient instructed to close firmly into retruded contact. When there is difficulty in accurately placing the paper, specially designed holders are available. Contacts are marked and adjustments made to the marked spots to produce an even occlusion. The nature of the procedure is such that most cusp tips show faint contacts, with well marked contacts occurring between premature cusps and the opposing fossae.

Using articulating paper it is sometimes difficult to distinguish between marks caused by premature contacts and accidental contacts. Another technique has therefore become popular, namely the use of occlusal indicator wax. First, the green wax is luted to the occlusal surfaces of the maxillary denture. The wax was originally designed for occlusal adjustment of natural teeth, and to aid adhesion to wet tooth surfaces one side is coated with a water soluble film. No problems are experienced when bonding the wax to dry acrylic teeth and good results can be achieved with or without the film. After instructing the patient to close into retruded contact, any premature contacts—which appear as perforations or near perforations of the wax—are marked through the wax with the pencil provided. Marked contacts are adjusted after removing the wax and the procedure repeated with the other denture. Remember that in patients with little interalveolar space, "occlusal" contact can occur between the tuberosity and retromolar pad regions of the base, and these also require adjustment.

If a slight occlusal defect is present but there is no antero-posterior or lateral discrepancy in the intercuspal position and the mandibular buccal cusps occlude with the maxillary fossae, adjustments can be made in the mouth in two stages after using either of the above described materials for identification of premature contacts. Whichever is chosen, after closing into the retruded contact position, premature cusp contacts are identified and the opposing fossae deepened. Cusps are preserved at this stage in case they serve a supporting role in lateral excursions. Premature contacts are next marked in lateral excursions on each working and balancing side in turn, and if possible the high spots reduced in accordance with the BULL rule, *viz.* buccal upper cusps and lingual lower cusps. The rule is applied in order to preserve balancing contacts on the non-working side but is not applicable in cross-bites, and need not be followed too slavishly so

long as sufficient other contacts occur on the adjusted side to allow denture stability. Finally, antero-posterior balance is checked and smooth movement in protrusion ensured by adjustment of the distal slopes of the maxillary buccal cusps and the mesial slopes of the mandibular lingual cusps.

When a single prominent cusp is identified which prevents contact in the intercuspal position, it is not always wise to adopt the classical treatment of adjusting the occlusion by deepening the opposing fossa. If the premature contact is more than minimal the result may well be to produce a marked concavity in the adjusted surface into which the elongated cusp fits. Not only is antero-posterior balance lost but further prolonged occlusal adjustment has to be carried out to allow balanced articulation in lateral excursions. Instead, the offending cusp should be reduced and the remainder of the tooth recontoured to the opposing teeth.

In complete denture prosthodontics cross-bite occlusal relationships are common and are frequently a consequence of the different resorption patterns of the edentulous alveolar ridges. Whereas in the maxilla resorption is more pronounced buccally and labially, in the molar region of the mandible it is predominantly on the lingual side. A cross-bite in the molar region is the usual result of setting the mandibular molars in their mechanically most favourable position over the residual ridge. If, to prevent a cross-bite, the mandibular artificial teeth are set slightly on the lingual side of the ridge in their functionally correct position there is a danger that the resulting undercut in the lingual polished surface can act as a destablizing factor, hence the mechanically stable site is often preferred. The change to a reverse occlusal relationship then occurs in the premolar region and a reverse BULL rule can be applied beyond this point. When a class III jaw relationship is present, all the posterior teeth can be expected to have a reverse occlusal relationship. While schemes of occlusal adjustment can be attempted, it is often best to minimize potential difficulties by prescribing non-anatomical flat-cusped teeth at the registration stage, especially if there has been marked alveolar resorption.

Check record

Skilled operators claim to be able to correct discrepancies in the antero-posterior or lateral occlusal relationships by adjustments in the above manner using articulating paper or occlusal indicator wax. Before placing too much reliance on either of these methods of occlusal adjustment, it must be remembered that dentures are supported on compressible tissue and on occlusion will move slightly in relationship to the supporting alveolar bone. In the presence of deflecting contacts the degree of accuracy that can be achieved in the mouth is therefore limited. When an incorrect occlusal relationship has been recorded, it is more usual to make a check record or remount procedure and perform the occlusal adjustment on an articulator.

A check record is made when the occlusal surfaces of the dentures are related to one another by closure in the hinge axis position towards the retruded contact position, but before occlusal contact has occurred and before cuspal interference can cause a deviation from the retruded contact position. A number of materials can be used, including zinc oxide/eugenol pastes, silicone rubbers and softened wax. In general zinc oxide pastes and silicone rubber impression materials are too fluid to prevent cuspal contact between the two dentures unless

extreme care is taken. Wax works well if softened to the correct consistency, but although cheap tends to distort if used carelessly. Recently developed forms of silicone-based registration pastes are excellent, and after a rapid set are hard and stable. A small amount of silicone putty bonded with tray adhesive to the teeth of the mandibular denture is clean and resists knocks but takes a little while to set and can be spoiled by patient movement.

If wax is used, a double-thickness strip is softened and luted to the occlusal surface of the mandibular denture. Maintaining the softness of the wax, the dentures are inserted and the patient instructed to close into retruded contact. Although the patient will have been reminded to avoid actual contact, inspection of the indented surfaces when the dentures have been separated usually shows a point at which this has occurred. A strip of single-thickness softened wax is layered on top of the first and the process repeated, when it is usually successful. The dentures are relocated extraorally using the wax record, sealed together more permanently with a hot knife and mounted on an articulator by the technician. The best silicone-based registration pastes are extrusion-mixed and are dispensed directly as a 1 cm strip bilaterally on the occlusal surface of the mandibular denture. Silicone putty is very easy to use but only those types which can have their speed of set increased by adding extra catalyst are useful. (Fig. 7.2).

Once the dentures are rigidly related to one another they can be adjusted on the articulator using the thinnest possible articulating paper to identify interferences, using the techniques described above. The technique of check record or remount procedure is of proven benefit in reducing subsequent patient discomfort[4] and using it, it is often possible to

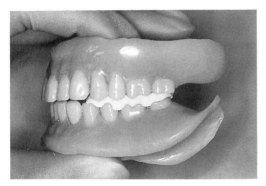

Fig. 7.2 Check record performed using silicone putty as locating material.

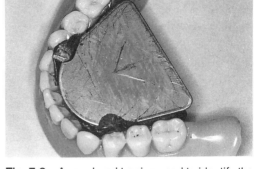

Fig. 7.3 Arrow-head tracing used to identify the retruded contact position when making a check record.

rectify quite gross occlusal faults and even provide moderate decreases in the occlusal face height.

Methods of greater complexity are also available for preparing check records. One involves a special zinc oxide/eugenol paste, but direct occlusal contact is prevented by interposing a preformed linen strip supported on a metal frame. Alternatively, if the equipment is available, a gothic arch or arrow-head tracing can be performed at a sufficiently increased face height to avoid cuspal interferences in lateral excursions. The plates are attached with composition to the appropriate dentures and the lower plate coated with wax pencil. After tracing an arrow-head on the waxed plate (Fig. 7.3) the tracing pointer is located over the apex by means of a perforated disc and sticky wax. Plaster keys in the molar region act to stabilize the arrangement before it is mounted on an articulator and occlusal adjustment performed as before.

Persistent pain

Although pain immediately on insertion of the dentures is easily treated, pain from the denture-bearing area which re-

mains even after occlusal adjustment, is often diffuse in character and the sources difficult to pin-point. Two materials, disclosing wax and pressure indicating paste, are available to aid their detection.

Disclosing wax

The technique for using disclosing wax is simple and the materials cheap. A small amount of wax is melted in a pot. When entirely liquid, it is applied in a thin layer with a stiff artist's paint brush to the entire fitting surface of the denture. Next, the smooth surface of the set wax is furrowed with the tip of the brush. After occluding firmly, pressure points show as flattening and perforation of the furrowed wax surface and are relieved (Fig. 7.4). If pain is still present the technique can be repeated and the surface adjusted again after removing surplus wax from the denture with a nailbrush and hot water.

Disclosing wax is also useful when inserting immediate or transitional overdentures to perfect the functional contact between the denture and the abutments. There is always an inaccurate fit between the surfaces of abutments which have been prepared in the mouth and the corresponding points of an overdenture

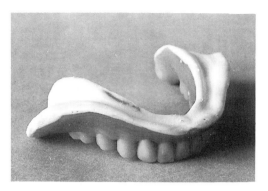

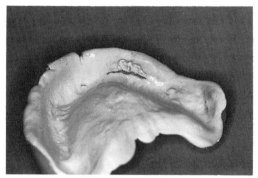

Fig. 7.4 Pressure spot in mandibular left lingual region revealed by use of disclosing wax.

Fig. 7.5A Perforations in pressure indicating paste identify areas of excess pressure. The mucosal defect apical to the main defect is caused by a small area of osteo-radionecrosis.

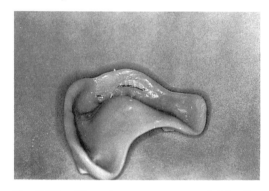

Fig. 7.5B Sites of excess pressure visible after removal of pressure indicating paste.

which has been processed to a prepared model. High spots on the base over the abutments are first identified with disclosing wax then removed. Subsequently, after coating the abutments with petroleum jelly which acts as a separating medium, autopolymerizing acrylic is placed on the fitting surface and when it has reached a dough stage the denture is seated under moderate occlusal pressure before cure is completed in a hydroflask. Any set resin which has been forced over other parts of the fitting surface or into the gingival crevice is removed and subsequently the fit of the denture will be optimal under load when the root abutments are brought into function.

Disclosing wax may come in an aerosol formulation and is sprayed onto the dried surface of the denture. While the method is quick and convenient, adhesion between the denture base and the applied paste is poor. The results can be messy and ambiguous unless extreme care is taken.

Pressure indicating paste

An alternative to disclosing wax is pressure indicating paste, which is a silicone paste similar in consistency to a fluid silicone impression material. After mixing a small amount—which is dispensed as base and catalyst from two tubes—it is spread over the fitting surface of the denture, the denture reinserted and the patient advised to close, first gently and then more firmly, into occlusion. The paste sets quickly, when the denture can be removed from the patient's mouth and the layer of paste inspected for perforations. The denture is marked with a fibre-tipped pen through each perforation and after the layer of silicone has been removed the fitting surface of the denture is relieved over the marks (Fig. 7.5A and B).

Nausea

If nausea has not been a problem with previous dentures and was not encountered during the impression stage, then if it occurs at this stage it is caused by intolerance of the new denture. Frequently the patient complains of the maxillary denture extension over their hard palate. If the extension is now greater than previously, nausea can be improved by reducing the posterior extension to the same extent as before. This eliminates the post dam, if one has been processed in, and a functional post dam must be made. However, with a post dam which is now partly sited over less compressible tissue, adequate retention is more difficult to achieve. A better treatment is to thin down the posterior edge of the palate to a knife-edge, making it less intrusive to the tongue. The patient is encouraged to habituate to this new situation by wearing the denture for increasingly longer periods during the day, but giving encouragement by making him aware of the increased retention now achieved with a properly extended palate and the poorer retention which will result if it has to be reduced. Reassurance must also be given that should your plan fail, a reduction of the posterior extension can be easily made.

Alternatively, nausea may be caused by an increase in bulk of the new dentures. This is common in the elderly and is indicative of the decreasing tolerance that the elderly have to comparatively small changes. Usually the patient can identify the problem site immediately and reduction of the bulk is a simple procedure, but at other times alterations to the position of teeth are required. It is then easier to begin again, but to avoid risking further disappointment, use a duplication procedure. Sometimes the increased bulk of the denture is part and parcel of an increased face height and if this error has been missed the patient's complaint of nausea will only be the preamble to numerous complaints at subsequent visits. Hence, also check at this stage that face height is correct. If an error is discovered it is usually easier to remake the mandibular denture to the correct vertical dimension.

Finally, the nausea felt by the patient might be symptomatic of lack of retention. Rectifying the fault in retention by placing a functional post dam or extending the periphery correctly will bring relief.

Denture identification

At this stage it again becomes necessary to consider whether denture identification is needed. Identification can be useful if it is thought that the patient is likely to spend a period of time in a hospital or nursing home, and is invaluable for forensic purposes and after accidents.[5] While a good case can be made for always providing some form of denture identification, it is best to ensure that patients give their consent before implementing the procedure. Many think it macabre and might have personal reasons for its rejection.

If an identification strip has not been incorporated in the denture during processing, then at this stage an identification code (often the initials or first five or six letters of the patient's name plus their postal code) can be simply applied by means of a spirit-based fibre-tipped pen, the mark being protected by a sealant. First, a section of each denture is chosen which is less likely to undergo abrasion—usually the buccal flange. A small area is dried, roughened with fine sandpaper and marked with a fine black pen. To improve the longevity of the marking two or more layers of clear sealant are placed over it with a brush and allowed to dry thoroughly. Proprietary kits are available, but the equipment can be prepared in the clinic, sealant being made by dissolving shavings of clear acrylic resin in chloroform.[6] While much cheaper than proprietary materials, the convenience of not having to make up the sealant outweighs the extra cost of the ready made kit unless the procedure is being used frequently.

The longevity of methods involving pens and sealant is not great and the marking has to be repeated at intervals of a few months. A more permanent way is to engrave the code figures into the denture with the tip of a scalpel. Rubbing the marks with a graphite pencil makes the lines more visible, following which a sealant is applied.[7] The method is less aesthetic because only digital-style figures, composed of straight lines, can be used.

An identification strip can be incorporated into a denture after processing by cutting a groove, placing the strip, then covering it with clear autopolymerizing acrylic. The identification strip is permanent but may act as a point of weakness or porosity. The process of making and inserting the identification strip takes extra time, which may be costly, and visibility is ultimately affected because the overlying autopolymerizing acrylic will fog with time.[8]

References

1. Becker, C.M., Smith, D.E. and Nicholls, J.I. The comparison of denture base processing techniques. Part II. Dimensional changes due to processing. *J Prosthet Dent* **37**:450–459, 1977.
2. Miller, T.H. Obtaining the posterior palatal seal. *J Prosthet Dent* **53**:717–718, 1984.
3. McCartney, J.W. Flange adaptation discrepancy, palatal base distortion, and induced malocclusion caused by processing acrylic resin maxillary complete dentures. *J Prosthet Dent* **52**:545–553, 1984.
4. Firtell, D.N., Finzen, F.C. and Holmes, J.B. The effect of clinical remount procedures on the comfort and success of complete dentures. *J Prosthet Dent* **57**:53–57, 1987.
5. Ayton, F.D., Hill, C.M. and Parfitt, H.N. The dental role in the identification of victims in the Bradford City football ground fire. *Br Dent J* **159**:262–265, 1985.
6. Heath, J.R., Zoitopoulos, L. and Griffiths, C. Simple methods for denture identification: a clinical trial. *J Oral Rehabil* **15**:587–592, 1988.
7. Stevenson, R.B. Marking dentures for identification. *J Prosthet Dent* **58**:255, 1987.
8. Fletcher, A.M., Turner, C.H. and Ritchie, G.M. Denture marking methods and induced stress. *Br Dent J* **142**:224–226, 1977.

Chapter 8

Review

Although we make every effort to eliminate sources of pain or dissatisfaction at the stage of denture delivery, it is impossible to be prescient enough to eliminate all possible sources and approximately 50% of our patients have a complaint later. For this reason the review visit should never be omitted. Whether it takes place after 24 hours or, as is often the case, after a week, it is consoling to patients (and perhaps helps them bear any discomfort with more fortitude) if they know they have a review appointment and that they are welcome back at the surgery should pain make their immediate attendence necessary. For the same reason they are reassured that their prosthodontist is a professional, caring person of integrity, when even after any problems have been eliminated at the review visit, they have been asked to return again should further correction be neeeded.

The problems that arise at the review stage are relatively few in number but at times can tax our diagnostic skill. Chief among them is pain, followed by lack of retention or instability. Less frequently patients complain of poor speech, clicking teeth or functional disturbances such as inability to eat. A complaint of poor appearance may arise if patients have been insufficiently consulted during the tooth selection stage or have not been allowed time to make up their minds at the try-in stage. Sometimes an indefinite dissatisfaction conceals a disappointment with the appearance which can only be unearthed be sensitive questioning. If nausea occurs at this stage as an entirely new complaint a fresh reason must be sought for its presence. Finally, the opportunity should be taken at this stage to assess patients' oral hygiene, and provide advice if needed.

Pain

When a patient attends at the review stage with a complaint of pain, diagnosis can be simplified by first categorizing the source of the pain. Generally pain is limited to one of four sites, the TMJ region, the lips and cheeks, the tongue, or most frequently the denture-bearing area.

Pain from the TMJ region

Pain in the temporomandibular joint region is usually associated with an error in the maxillo-mandibular relationships, usually a lack of freeway, or interocclusal space. Pain from this region is then often overlayed by simultaneous pain from the mandibular denture-bearing area, but in cases where an attempt has previously been made to eliminate pain by modifying the fitting surface of the denture with a soft liner the pain from the TMJ region may be the presenting symptom. Once the cause has been confirmed by careful measurement of the rest face height and occlusal face height, there is little that can be done apart from replacing the offending denture. Pain in the TMJ region as a consequence of decreased face height is unusual at the review stage and normally only occurs after prolonged wear without professional recall. It might even be questioned whether a reduction in face height predisposes to TMJ pain. When comparing two edentulous populations, one wearing dentures and one without, TMJ pain was found to be less common in the latter, where overclosure would have been maximal.[1]

Cheek and lip biting

When freeway space is excessive a more likely site for pain than the TMJ region is the cheek, the mucosa of the cheek tending to be trapped in the enlarged interocclusal space until new habits of muscle control are learned. When the complaint persists the operator should check that there is adequate bucco-lingual occlusal overjet. Where the bucco-lingual occlusal relationships are also normal, i.e. there is no cross-bite, cheek and lip biting is always caused by a lack of anterior or posterior overjet and it can often be corrected in the mouth by slightly reducing the buccal surfaces of the buccal cusps of mandibular posterior teeth or the labial surfaces of mandibular anterior teeth, followed by careful repolishing.

Complications occur when the posterior teeth are in a cross-bite relationship or the anterior teeth in an edge-to-edge relationship. In the former case the dentures should be related to one another in the intercuspal position, mounted on an articulator, and individual adjustments made by the operator. When a cross-bite exists the teeth causing the problem are usually those at the point where the change from positive to negative overjet occurs and the only solution is to reduce the occlusal surfaces of both buccal cusps out of contact with one another.

When lip biting is associated with an edge-to-edge incisor relationship, adjustment is more difficult. Sometimes by careful alteration of the facets on the incisal edges a slight degree of overjet can be made and at the same time incisal contact still maintained in protrusion. When this does not cure the problem, the mandibular incisors have to be removed, a new set waxed to the base in a retroclined position, and permanently secured after a try-in. The mandibular incisors are replaced for preference partly because an addition around the mandibular teeth is less obvious, but primarily because the maxillary incisors play a major part in the support of the upper lip and interference with their position might cause problems with appearance or speech.

Pain from the tongue

There are two possible denture-related causes for this problem, either direct trauma to the tongue or restriction of its movement. If traumatic in origin it may be caused by a rough or irregular lingual surface and is easily cured either by polishing any rough surfaces identified by the patient, or removing the irregularities, which are usually the result of an attempt by the technician to produce a natural gingival margin for the lingual surfaces of the teeth. On the other hand, the pain may be located at the tip of the tongue and be related to a diastema which the patient has asked to be incorporated but which irritates the tongue. To eliminate the source of irritation but at the same time preserve appearance, the diastema is filled with clear, autopolymerizing acrylic resin.

The other possible cause is that the posterior teeth may have been set too far lingually and lack of space is causing cramping of the tongue. The pain resulting is not acute but is described as a diffuse burning sensation, relieved when the denture is left out. The condition can be suspected if the lateral border of the tongue shows indentations caused by the teeth and confirmed by comparing with dividers the tongue space present on the offending dentures with that present on a previous set of satisfactory dentures.

When little extra space is required and the occlusion permits it, the lingual cusps can be trimmed from the mandibular teeth to provide more space. When this is not enough, new complete dentures must be made. A previous satisfactory denture is usually available for comparison and the amount of tongue space can be reproduced. If despite adequate tongue space the pain is still present, or if it is otherwise suspected that the trouble is not denture-related, further treatment can be prescribed as for that of "burning mouth" syndrome in Chapter 1.

Pain from the denture-bearing surface

Diagnosis of the cause of pain from the denture-bearing surface can be difficult. Before initiating any treatment it should be determined by close examination and palpation whether the painful area is peripheral or central, diffuse or discrete, and whether or not associated with an area of erythema. Armed with these facts, diagnosis and treatment are straightforward. Temporary soft linings will successfully relieve pain of this nature—even that caused by excessive face height, despite increasing the face height even further—but they have no place in the diagnosis and are no substitute for adequate assessment.

Pain at the periphery of the denture-bearing area, when associated with an area of erythema, is caused by overextension of the associated denture. If an overextension involves a muscle attachment and if the intrinsic retention of the denture is good the overextension will cause pain. When retention is poor, overextension interferes with muscle function and the patient's complaint will be one of looseness of the denture, which will be dealt with below. The commonest sites in the lower jaw for a complaint of pain uncomplicated by a complaint of looseness, are over the external oblique ridge, over unnoticed lingual tori, and over the mylohyoid ridge, the latter being difficult to see and hence easily missed. In the maxilla the common sites of pain are over the post dam or in the distal tuberosity region.

Occasionally, pain at the disto-buccal edge of the mandibular denture is felt only when patients occlude their teeth. It is then caused by pressure of the contracted masseter muscle against the denture. Impressions are normally taken with the mouth open and the masseter muscles displaced relatively backwards by the movement of the head of the condyle downwards and forwards. On occlusion the condyles move distally and the contracted masseters contact the disto-buccal extension of any mandibular denture made with an open-mouth impression technique. In a similar way, if impressions have been made with a closed-mouth technique, pain may be caused in the tuberosity region on opening the mouth. Then the pain is caused by pressure of the coronoid process as it moves forwards and comes into contact with the buccal flange of the maxillary denture.

Treatment is always preceded by precise localization of the part of the denture which causes the pain. After drying the mucosa, a small amount of the zinc oxide component of zinc oxide/eugenol impression paste is placed with a blunt probe on the painful site. The denture is inserted, the paste transfers itself to the area of overextension and the marked spot is reduced. When it is suspected that the coronoid process is involved, the extension of the flange lying buccal to the tuberosity is thinned. An excessively deep post dam can be reduced, but with care to avoid loosing retention. Palatal overextension onto the mobile part of the soft palate produces similar symptoms to those of excessive post dam but is more uncommon. The line of redness resembles that produced by an excessive post dam but will recur unless, after confirming the overextension by palpation of the junction of hard and soft palate, the extension of the palate is reduced back to this point and a functional post dam added using autopolymerizing acrylic.

In the absence of an obvious undercut, pain and redness of the central part of the denture-bearing surface can have a variety of causes. Much can be diagnosed from its appearance. If it diffusely but unevenly covers much of the mandibular denture-bearing surface the cause is probably lack of interocclusal space and checking the jaw relationships will confirm the diagnosis. Very rarely, a diffuse painful area covering the entire denture-bearing surface and extending onto the cheeks is associated with allergy, but before concluding that an allergy to acrylic resin is present it is sensible to rather suspect the presence of excess monomer in the denture and contact the technician for details of the processing technique employed. Alternatively, if only

the maxillary denture-bearing area is affected and pain is minimal, denture stomatitis is the likely cause.

Differential diagnosis between denture stomatitis and allergy can be made by first taking swabs to confirm or exclude candidosis. In the absence of other signs of acrylic allergy (e.g. scaling lesions where spectacle frames or acrylic textiles touch the skin) it is possible to perform skin sensitivity tests oneself but it is probably best to refer the patient to a dermatologist. An undisputed diagnosis of sensitivity to acrylic polymer or monomer may then be made, if necessary by lymphocyte transformation tests.[2]

Large, but less extensive, red, painful areas beneath the mandibular denture may be the consequence of a thin, friable mucosa or insufficient saliva—sometimes both—usually involving an elderly individual. Apart from prescribing an artificial saliva or advising the use of a small amount of denture adhesive to act as a lubricant, there is little that can be done. Many cases of hyposalivation are associated with drug therapy, usually for cardio-vascular problems or depression, and if artificial saliva gives relief it would seem pointless to interfere with the patient's medication if it is proving effective. When the mucosa of an elderly individual is thin, tender and friable it is tempting to provide a resilient liner, but this form of treatment should be avoided if possible. If the friable mucosa is associated with insufficient saliva and a silicone liner is prescribed, the increased coefficient of friction between the liner and the dry mucosa will make the problem worse.

The commonest reason for a moderately large, diffuse area of pain and redness, on the denture-bearing surface is a problem with the occlusion. It is most usually associated with the mandibular denture-bearing surface because there the abnormal stresses resulting from the occlusal fault have a smaller area of support, and tissue overloading is more likely. Try first to identify the most likely cause, which is a premature occlusal contact, and then measure the vertical jaw relations carefully, searching for an unnoticed increase in occlusal face height. Finally, investigate the possibility of a discrepancy between the retruded contact position and the intercuspal position.

When single premature contacts are found they can be removed by adjustment of the occlusal surface with a stone in the same way as described at the denture-delivery stage, and when discrepancies between the intercuspal position and the retruded contact position are identified, a check record is made. Lack of freeway space means that it is necessary to replace the mandibular denture unless the vertical discrepancy is very slight, when a reduction in face height by means of a check record can be tried.

A small, red, discrete, painful area is of simple aetiology, and if after careful examination of the area there is no sign of a sinus or retained root and radiographic examination proves negative, the cause is invariably a defect of the fitting surface of the denture. The area at fault can be located by means of a small amount of zinc oxide paste in the same way as areas of overextension are identified. When the painful spot is on the most prominent buccal or labial part of the alveolar ridge the cause is usually an unnoticed undercut and that part of the denture base entering the undercut zone should be relieved. When over the central area of the palate it is usually due to the presence of a palatine torus, the thin mucoperiosteum providing insufficient cushioning from the forces of mastication. In the event that neither can be identified, close examination of the suspect area of the denture-base will reveal

an area of roughness caused by damage to the model prior to processing or an unnoticed pimple of acrylic where, under the pressure of flasking, acrylic has been forced into a subsurface void in the plaster.

In all cases where the fitting surface is to be adjusted with a small stone or bur, removal of acrylic should be minimal. Stop as soon as the pain is relieved. Because there is redness of the affected site there must be swelling which will resolve when the stimulus is removed. Disclosing wax is not to be used otherwise the swollen tissues might displace the wax excessively and lead to unnecessary reduction of the base. Where the base has been reduced the roughened area is finally smoothed with pumice.

Sometimes the area of pain may be promptly identified by the patient and be sensitive to palpation but show no evidence of erythema. The two common sites for this are in the region of the mental foramen where resorption has resulted in the foramen lying superficially on the crest of the ridge, and in the mandibular anterior region when resorption has been irregular and sharp bony spicules remain which cause pain from the overlying tissue when the patient chews.

In the case of a superficial mental foramen, generous relief of the denture over the area, at the chairside, is the only satisfactory treatment. When sharp bony spicules are present on the crest of the ridge beneath the mucoperiosteum and adjusting the fitting surface does not provide relief, surgical reduction is the ideal treatment (Fig. 8.1) but in the event that the patient is frail or otherwise unsuitable for surgery, a resilient liner may be the last (and not always successful) resort. There are two types, silicone rubber and plasticized poly (ethyl methacrylate) resins, neither of which can be said to be permanent. The former will require replacement after about a year following

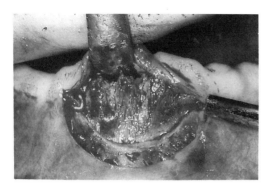

Fig. 8.1 Bone spicule of anterior mandibular alveolus revealed at operation.

failure of the adhesive bond between the lining and the denture base, and the latter after about the same time following hardening of the lining after leaching out of the plasticizer. Experienced clinicians tend to avoid prescribing resilient liners. The patient quickly becomes accustomed to having a resilient liner, will prove difficult to wean off it in the future, and will demand a similar replacement each time.

In the event that it does become necessary it is still possible to add a resilient liner at this stage. After removing any undercuts from the fitting surface, an impression is taken with a fluid silicone of either the addition or condensation-cure type. A model is cast and the technician removes at least 2 mm from the fitting surface of the denture to allow an adequate thickness of lining. Controversy exists whether it is better to box-in the lining or whether the periphery should be left free. Boxed-in linings may have a better prognosis for retention but enclosing them makes them less soft.[3] The technical stages for a boxed lining are also more difficult, and part of the boxing is so often lost after having to reduce the periphery that the real advantages are minimal.

The fitting surface of a plasticized poly (ethyl methacrylate) resilient liner is eas-

ily adjusted with normal equipment, but silicone linings are a problem, and are difficult to trim with any item of conventional equipment apart from a scalpel. Fortunately, special stones and burs have been developed which give a very satisfactory result.

Retention and stability

At this point it is important to re-emphasize the necessity for adequate diagnosis. All too often a complaint of looseness by the patient is followed by provision of a permanent reline for the offending denture without adequate diagnosis of the fault. Unless the cause of the "looseness" has been correctly identified, arbitrary treatment of this nature will lead only to even greater patient dissatisfaction.

Patients often complain of looseness of their dentures and only a perceptive patient will distinguish between lack of retention and instability. First take a history and distinguish between the two types of complaint. Generally, if the denture is loose to a direct pull upwards or downwards a retention fault can be suspected, while if the patient complains of looseness but the dentures resist a direct pull, lack of stability is the cause of the complaint. Again, if the patient complains of looseness only when eating and speaking—but particularly when speaking—a fault of stability is likely. Dentures loose at all times indicate a retention fault.

Retention

A complete denture in position, separated by a thin film of saliva from the underlying tissues, is displaced when sufficient force is applied to cause shearing of the saliva film. The integrity of the saliva film is maintained by the intermolecular forces of adhesion and cohesion, forces which at the macroscopic level are measurable as viscosity. Drawing analogies with the parallel plate situation, the retention of a complete denture is greatest under three conditions, namely when the area of the fitting surface is maximal but not so great as to cause muscle interference, when the apposition between the denture and the mucosa is as close as possible, and when the saliva possesses optimum viscosity. Although a retention fault may be diagnosed as being either physiological, anatomical, clinical or technical in origin, each fault must diminish retention by the extent to which it fails to fulfill the above conditions.

Rarely, patients will complain of lack of retention despite all efforts to improve it, their complaint being that "the upper denture tilts down at the back when I bite". If questioned, such patients will demonstrate the fault themselves and in doing so show that they make no attempt to control the maxillary denture with their tongue—the tongue remaining on the floor of the mouth when incising. The lack of muscular control that is shown is sometimes a result of ignorance, and simple instructions will improve matters. Unfortunately it can also be due to an inadequate personality, the patient enjoying the disability and the attention it provokes.

Physiological fault

Check first that there is adequate saliva and that the mucosa is not dry. In the absence, or relative absence, of saliva the fitting surface of the denture will not be covered by an intact film of saliva and retention will suffer. It has been shown that although degenerative changes in the salivary glands occur with age even in healthy patients, in the parotid at least this is not reflected by a significant reduction in either stimulated or resting flow rates.[4] The cause of hyposalivation is almost invariably drug therapy. Consequently, apart from advising the sucking of citrus sweets or the prescribing of an artificial saliva there is little that can be done if the medication is to be continued. When in cases of hyposalivation an artificial saliva is prescribed, the increase in retention is dramatic because some of the ingredients which are added to improve the lubrication qualities (e.g. sodium carboxymethyl cellulose, polyethylene oxide etc.) are those used by manufacturers to make denture adhesives.

Anatomical fault

If substantial alveolar undercuts are present the denture base has to be relieved from the undercuts to allow easy placement. This produces either a local thickening of the saliva film which is sheared more easily or else the integrity of the film is destroyed by the presence of an air bubble. In either case retention is worse and to compensate for the lack of retention a facial seal has to be established. This is relatively easy labially where the facial muscles are firmly applied to a normally extended labial flange but in the buccal region it is necessary to thicken the periphery to achieve a functional seal with the buccal mucosa. Ideally an impression is made in zinc oxide/eugenol or silicone supported by composition or silicone putty and an addition made in heat-cured acrylic resin. An immediate addition can be made in cold-cure resin, but porosity can occur and the presence of residual monomer is a potential disadvantage.

The precise site for the addition is a source of controversy. Some say that the thickening should be in the deepest part of the sulcus so that pressure is applied to the insertions of the muscles in a lateral direction. Others say that the form of the thickening should resemble the anatomical shape of the alveolar bone which has been lost and therefore advise that the thickening should be further onto the polished surface, the periphery remaining as more of a knife-edge. Both forms produce adequate retention.

Clinical fault

Despite adequate saliva and lack of undercuts, use of a poor clinical technique can still cause loss of peripheral seal, most often in the post dam region. To diagnose the site the denture is held in place then tilted forwards, backwards and from side to side. Loss of retention with a forwards tilt indicates lack of a post dam, and loss of retention to tilting in other directions indicates lack of peripheral or facial seal, the site being indicated by the direction of the tilt which causes displacement. Small additions to the post dam or periphery can be made by the techniques outlined above or in previous chapters.

Difficulties are encountered when the post dam has been sited too far anteriorly and is attempting to form a functional seal with incompressible tissue over the midline of the palate. Additions are made to the distal of the denture with Greenstick composition or functional trim material until it is extended to the correct site. A localized impression is made with a fluid impression material, either zinc oxide/eugenol or silicone. A model is cast and an addition made. A functional post dam is added in the surgery after the extension is complete.

Technical fault

Uncompensated polymerization shrinkage can lead to a poorly fitting denture base. This is most often encountered in the case of the maxillary denture when shrinkage of the resin pulls the unpolymerized dough away from the fitting surface of the palate.[5] Careful additions to the periphery will improve the retention, but when shrinkage is marked the patient is aware that the base of the denture is a poor fit and will complain of lack of central contact. A new denture must be made.

Stability

When a problem of instability has been diagnosed, examine each of the surfaces of the faulty denture in turn. The fitting surface, occlusal/incisal surface and polished surface may each be responsible and defects in their form must be eliminated before the blame can be placed on an anatomical, physiological or pathological condition.

Fitting surface

If the fitting surface of the denture encroaches on the insertion of a muscle, the denture will be unstable when the muscle contracts unless it is particularly retentive, when the presenting symptom will be pain. To identify the muscle responsible, the relationship of each of the major muscles attached around the periphery of the denture should be studied in turn. With the mandibular denture in place and held down by the operator's finger tips, the patient is requested to touch their soft palate with the tip of their tongue. Displacement of the denture against finger pressure indicates overextension in the midline over the genioglossus muscle. Subsequently, touching the right and left commissures with the tongue indicates overextension over the left and right mylohyoid muscles, respectively. Finally, protrusion of the tongue may cause displacement of the denture and points to an overextension distally of the disto-lingual flange into the path of movement of the palatoglossus.

To examine the relationships of the buccal musculature to the mandibular denture, the modiolus should be grasped and drawn first backwards and inwards and then forwards and inwards, feeling for denture movement caused by overextension over the insertions of the buccinator and the depressor muscles of the lower lip. Finally, by taking hold of the lower lip in the midline and raising it any interference with the mentalis muscle can be detected. If the patient subsequently claims that movement of the denture follows normal contraction of the mentalis muscle—as in a pouting-like action—overextension anteriorly is confirmed.

Testing for overextension of the maxillary denture is simpler. If the denture is displaced by drawing the modiolus downwards and forwards, an extension is indicated over the insertion of the buccinator into the maxilla. Drawing the modiolus downwards and back will test for an extension of the labial flange over the insertion of the upper lip muscles. While the minor slips of the orbicularis oris which insert into the maxilla and define the depth of the anterior sulcus can be tested by drawing the upper lip down manually, it is probably easier to allow the patient to perform the movement themselves. Observe any displacement of the denture which occurs when the patient purses their lips and protrudes them in a pouting action.

If an overextension is detected the denture is relieved over the appropriate muscle. This is done gradually, questioning the patient on the degree of improvement, in order to ensure that maximum stable extension is retained.

Occlusal/incisal surface

All occlusal defects should have been corrected at an earlier stage, if a check record or remount procedure has been carried out, but when patients wear dentures for the first time, or after a prolonged period of wearing a faulty denture, their habitual jaw relationships can still be effective and it can then be argued that it is better to leave the check record until the review stage when the faulty reflexes have had the opportunity of being lost when the occlusal fault can then reveal itself in a complaint of looseness which is eliminated after a check record. It can be further argued that when placing dentures on a denture-bearing area which shows areas of erythema due to previous illfitting appliances, some resolution of inflammation may occur during the post-insertion phase. Here too the changes in the denture-bearing area may reveal themselves as previously unnoticed occlusal defects and looseness and may be corrected by a check record at the review stage.

In the same way as at the insertion stage, occlusal adjustment can sometimes be made in the mouth. If a premature contact is present the symptom will be tipping of the denture. Premature contacts can be detected with articulating paper and reduced following the rules outlined in the previous chapter. Unless the premature contact is large—and at this stage it is unlikely—a deepening of the opposing fossa is the treatment required.

A slight discrepancy in coincidence of intercuspal position and retruded contact position is fairly common following the patient's habituation to their new dentures and the relaxation which accompanies familiarity. As before, the patient's complaint will be of instability of the denture, most often the mandibular because the excellent retention of the maxillary denture resists displacing forces. When an intercuspal/retruded contact discrepancy is detected, a check record is performed.

Instability of the mandibular denture at this stage may also be due to a relative lack of interocclusal space, with cuspal interference between the near-contacting occlusal surfaces causing instability during speaking. Usually the interocclusal space can be increased slightly by means of a check record and stability improved —especially if high cusped teeth have been prescribed and the opportunity is taken of producing a less prominent cusp form. A similar type of instability may be present when a patient with atrophic ridges is given dentures with prominent cusps. Interference between the cusps will cause a complaint of instability even when a balanced articulation is produced. Again a reduction of the cusp heights in conjunction with a check record or remount procedure is the treatment of choice.

Although when dealing with denture stability most textbooks cite the need to lower the occlusal plane so that the body of the tongue overlaps the mandibular occlusal surface, it is not often that instability of a mandibular denture can be attributed to an excessively high occlusal plane. Nevertheless, it must not be overlooked and in marginal cases the site of the occlusal surfaces in the vertical plane may affect stability.

With a few qualifications, dentures are most stable when the artificial teeth occupy the same positions as they did in life. One exception is when after a prolonged period of not wearing a complete denture, with consequent tongue spreading, the most stable positon for the teeth is further buccal than expected. With teeth set in the anatomically correct position and this type of past dental history,

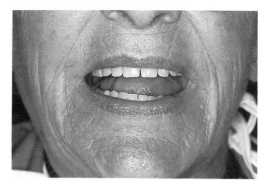

Fig.8.2 Mandibular denture lifts on right on opening the mouth. The mandibular incisors are set too far labially and act as a displacing factor.

although a patient may complain that the dentures are loose when speaking but function satisfactorily when eating, he is more likely to complain of general discomfort. A neutral zone record can be helpful in relocating the mandibular teeth in a more stable site.

The other exception occurs if, when placing the mandibular molars in their correct site, an undercut of the lingual polished surface is produced. Instability when speaking is again the complaint. Some degree of compromise may be made by reducing the bucco-lingual thickness of the posterior teeth at the expense of their lingual cusps, when the extra space created might eliminate the undercut and provide sufficient tongue space for comfortable speaking. It is important that this operation is explained to the patient, otherwise the mutilation of "their" denture and its subsequent altered appearance might provoke antagonism.

Instability may also occur if the incisal surfaces of the teeth have been set in error in an unstable position, and a new denture must be made with attention paid to placing the teeth in their pre-extraction sites. A common fault is to allow the mandibular anterior teeth to lie too far labially in order to permit a near normal overjet for a skeletal class II patient. The denture typically becomes loose immediately the patient opens their mouth or on smiling (Fig. 8.2). It is also a common error to misjudge the amount of resorption which has taken place in the maxillary anterior region and place the maxillary incisors insufficiently far labially, but unless the retention of the maxillary denture is poor, instability is rarely complained of. In class III cases destabilizing lingually directed pressure may come in the mandibular premolar region from the modiolus and can be resisted by setting the maxillary premolar teeth further buccally.

Polished surface

It is said to be advantageous to have a generally concave polished surface with the exceptions that the mandibular buccal polished surface can be made convex to permit it to conform to the buccinator muscle and prevent food accumulation, and if a neutral zone impression technique is performed, the lingual polished surface in the mandibular anterior region sometimes protrudes as a shelf. In practice, this aspect of the denture form is determined by the site of the functional periphery, the activity of the circumoral muscles, and the positioning of the occlusal and incisal surfaces of the teeth. If this permits a concave polished surface to be established then we should consider ourselves fortunate.

When the shape of the polished surface is such as to cause instability, patients will not only complain of looseness of the denture but can sometimes direct the operator to the particular part requiring attention. Where the mandibular polished surface in the posterior lingual region is too thick, the patient will additionally complain specifically of interference between this area of the denture and the tongue.

At other times the defect will be more difficult to pin down but two particular cases should be investigated when an otherwise satisfactory mandibular denture is unstable during speech. If the lingual polished surface is undercut in relation to the tongue, then the mechanical interference during speech results in denture movement. Alternatively, the instability can be a consequence of interference with the movements of the modiolus. Such defects in the polished surface are a consequence of the bucco/lingual position of the occlusal surface and have been dealt with earlier under this heading.

Rarely, instability of the maxillary denture is caused by the coronoid process contacting an excessively thick buccal flange during opening. Pain on opening is the usual symptom, but may be masked by a destabilizing interference which can be the principal complaint.

Anatomical

At times even the most retentive denture will lack stability if the residual alveolar ridge is either very resorbed or very fibrous. If missed in the assessment stage and no warning given, precautions taken, or surgical treatment advised to limit instability, there is little that can be done apart from tendering one's apologies to the patient. Sometimes the instability will be a consequence of a prominent palatal torus, causing the maxillary denture to tip and flex during function. This should have been noted at the assessment stage and note made to relieve the denture at the insertion stage. In the event that preliminary adjustment has proved inadequate, further relief can be given by adjustment of the fitting surface.

Physiological

Habituation to new dentures by the elderly is slow and may never be complete. General, non-specific dissatisfaction should lead the practitioner to compare the shape of the polished surface with that of a previous satisfactory denture. When a previous satisfactory denture is available it is possible to get good results using a duplication technique, but when an elderly patient is rendered edentulous without having first experienced and habituated to a partial denture, the prognosis must be guarded. Transitional type dentures are of great value in such cases and their use is advised whenever possible.

Pathological

Some psychotropic drugs produce as a side effect spasmodic movements of the facial musculature and tongue (tardive dyskinesia).[6] While the patient's complaint of a loose denture is very real it is beyond the ability of the prosthodontist to cure. Similarly, neuromuscular disease—such as Parkinson's disease—can make control of a mandibular denture impossible and the limit of the prosthodontist's ability is to provide a retentive maxillary denture.

Nausea and retching

Retching is a frustrating complaint to come across and methods for combatting it have been reviewed recently.[7] It is sometimes made worse by a tendency to hypersalivation resulting from the reaction to a large foreign body in the mouth. Minor degrees of nausea are often met with at the denture delivery stage especially if, to improve retention, the bases have been extended further than pre-

viously. Usually the discomfort has been overcome by the review stage and patients have habituated themselves well to the alterations that have been made. If nausea is still present the patient's responses to three questions will reveal the nature of the problem and indicate the potential for improvement.

"Have you ever been able to wear dentures comfortably?" If the answer is "yes" then you must suspect your own handiwork. One of the commonest causes is lack of interocclusal space and the first task is to re-check the jaw relations. If a lack of interocclusal space is discovered the treatment is replacement of at least the mandibular denture. Alternatively, the cause might be a non-retentive maxillary denture, the nausea being caused by contact of the dropping denture with the dorsum of the tongue. Further questioning will reveal the associated complaint of lack of retention and this can be dealt with as described earlier. There may be intrusion into the tongue space as a consequence of excess bulk or when a neutral zone fault is present. Again, when dealing with the problem of excess bulk, examination of the previous denture will reveal whether the difference is significant and indicate the site for reduction. If it involves reduction of the extension of the palate of the maxillary denture, removal of the post-dam will cause loss of retention and the consequences have to be explained to the patient. When a satisfactory extension has been achieved a functional post-dam can be placed using autopolymerizing acrylic resin.

If the answer to the question is "no", treatment of the problem is more likely to be unsuccessful. Unless it has been recognized at the assessment stage or while making impressions, when a course of slow adaptation to a prosthesis can be planned, treatment is difficult. Relaxation and controlled breathing exercises

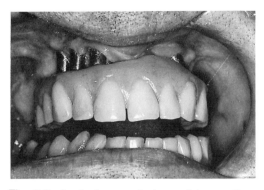

Fig. 8.3 Implant supported complete maxillary denture for patient with nausea.

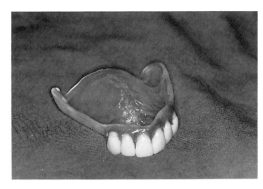

Fig. 8.4A Clear maxillary acrylic training base, with anteriors attached, for patient with nausea.

are helpful to many patients,[8] and where gradual adaptation fails, psychotherapy involving hypnosis or behavioral therapy can be tried. Both can sometimes achieve good results and a patient may be referred to a practitioner skilled in their dental application, but warned that treatment will be prolonged. If this form of therapy is unavailable and the patient believes that the nausea is a consequence of a lack of retention of the mandibular denture, implant supported dentures are now a final possibility (Fig. 8.3).

"Did you have the same problem when impressions were taken?" If the answer is "no" then the prognosis must be good and with a further period of habituation success will come about. Do not be tempted to reduce the palatal extension at the patient's demand. Instead the patient should be reassured and an appointment made for a month's time with the promise that you will be available for consultation during that time if required.

When the answer is "yes", but dentures have been worn previously, again the patient should habituate to the new dentures in time. If, however, the patient has not worn dentures before it now becomes necessary to attempt gradual habituation

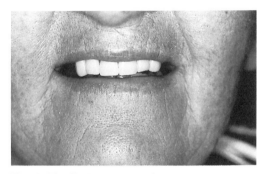

Fig. 8.4B Patient successfully wearing training base.

before reintroducing the patient to denture wear.

Impressions are taken, thin heat-cured acrylic bases are made and taken to the full extent of the denture-bearing area. Many patients find clear acrylic bases more tolerable. Perhaps they look less like dentures!

After carrying out any necessary adjustments to the extension for comfort, the patient wears the bases (first only the maxillary then also the mandibular) for increasing periods of time until they can be worn with comfort. The six maxillary anterior teeth are next added in wax to the base at the chairside to ensure that appearance is satisfactory. When the patient is satisfied, the teeth are attached permanently with autopolymerizing acrylic resin and a new period of habituation started (Fig. 8.4A and B). In turn, the mandibular anteriors, maxillary and mandibular premolars and, if possible, molars are added in a like fashion. Often, despite the best will of the patient, progress beyond the premolars proves impossible or if molars can be added their lingual cusps must be removed to reduce the space they occupy. In successful cases, when complete adaptation occurs the original dentures can be returned to the patient. When gradual habituation to a denture proves impossible despite supportive professional help, it is tempting to classify the problem as being of psychological origin, but psychotherapy is not always effective.

The final question is, "Is the nausea of recent onset?" If the answer is "yes" a systemic cause can be suspected. Nausea can complicate gastro-intestinal disease, and if suspected your suspicions should be immediately communicated to the patient's medical practitioner.

Poor speech

Patients usually adapt readily to moderate changes in denture shape, and problems with speech which are apparent at the delivery stage are not often present at the review. Adaptation occurs rapidly over the first few days, but if distortions of speech persist after 30 days a change to the denture has to be made. Remember, however, that adaptation of speech patterns back to normal is prolonged when the patient has a hearing impediment, and not all patients will admit to such a disability.[9]

Obstinate problems are of four types. Lack of interocclusal space produces difficulty with the fricative ("s" and "sh") and africative ("th") sounds. Because of the lack of room for proper articulation, speech is permanently sibilant, the patient often complaining that they sound drunk. Sibilance of speech may also be associated with a complaint of "clicking" of the dentures when speaking. The cause is the same—lack of interocclusal space—and can only be rectified by decreasing the face height. If the error is slight it may be possible to produce a sufficient increase by a check record or remount procedure. If more severe, new dentures must be made. An excellent test is for patients to read word couplets containing the difficult sounds, e.g. "fish-sheet" and "dish-cheese".[10]

An excessively thick palate will cause difficulty with plosive sounds, e.g. "ch", "ck" and "t". Adaptation is normally satisfactory with this type of fault, but thinning of the palate or even replacement of the denture by one with a metal base may sometimes be needed.

The most common problems arise when the anterior teeth are misplaced either anteriorly or posteriorly. Patients will clearly state the particular sounds they have difficulty with. When "f" and "v" sounds are faulty the site of the maxillary anterior teeth must be changed in the vertical plane, either to a higher or lower position. The lower lip has to make contact with these teeth during pronunciation of the sounds and if the sounds are difficult to make the site of the incisor edges must be raised. Conversely, excess hissing noise means that the incisors must be lowered. Problems with "th" sounds are again indicative of improperly sited maxillary anterior teeth, but this time in an incorrect antero-posterior position, to the extent that the tip of the tongue cannot achieve contact.

A complaint of general difficulty with speech can be associated with a lack of interocclusal space, but can also be caused by too low an occlusal plane or a decreased tongue space. The problem results from the more difficult manoeuvering required by the tongue to achieve normal speech. When severe, not only must a new denture have a higher occlusal plane but also more tongue space has to be created by setting the posterior teeth further buccally. The comfortable position of the teeth may need to be determined by means of a neutral zone record. Rarely a patient will complain of hissing when attempting to pronounce "l" sounds. The cause is excessive tongue space in the molar region and can be corrected by replacing the maxillary posterior teeth in a more lingual position.

Finally, interference with speech may be present in an elderly person without any obvious cause and it must be assumed that a prolonged period of adaptation to new dentures will be needed. Often the previous dentures have unusual jaw relationships, or excessive interocclusal space has resulted from resorption taking place over a prolonged period of time without denture replacement, or abnormal incisor relationships have been caused by protrusive overclosure. More satisfactory habituation to new dentures can be brought about by duplicating the previous dentures and incorporating only slight changes.

Denture fracture

When a patient returns at the review stage with a fractured denture it is important to determine first the cause of fracture before having it repaired. A history must be taken to discover the circumstances under which the fracture occurred, although the possibilities are more limited than when a similar history is taken at the assessment stage. At the review stage two types of fracture may be encountered—the accidental and the stress-induced. Dropping of the denture is a frequent occurrence for the accident prone or elderly and infirm. The denture can be repaired but permanent help can only be given by replacing the denture with one made from an impact resistant resin, when the rubber/acrylic co-polymer may be of help by preventing fracture propagation.

A denture fracturing under normal function, implies that normal function involves the application of stresses too great for the strength of acrylic resin to withstand and that a stress concentrating factor is present. The fractured surfaces must be examined for signs of porosity, lack of adhesion of the artificial teeth to the denture base, or evidence of previous fracture, and the mouth examined for anatomical features which might predispose to fracture such as undercuts, tori, or prominent ridges with little interalveolar space.

When physical defects of the base are visible, no denture repair can be expected to be permanent and to ensure that fracture does not occur again the denture has to be replaced, taking care over the processing to ensure that porosity does not occur, and by scrupulous cleanliness that adhesion between the base and teeth is optimized. In the meantime the denture has to be repaired temporarily and the patient warned that fracture might occur again.

In the absence of a fault in the denture base the strength of a repair bond approaches that of bulk resin. The most successful techniques for repair are therefore those which ensure that the surfaces to be joined are clean and have a large surface area available for bonding. Abrasion of the opposed surfaces with pumice is recommended. Any degree of lack of alignment will cause masticatory forces to stress the adhesive bond, making it more prone to further fracture, and if the repair is intended to last for any length of time, then to ensure that such forces are minimized a reline and check record should be performed.

Some patients are capable of fracturing all types of denture, and are exemplified by a person with large masseter muscles, a reduced interalveolar space and a stress concentrating factor such as a prominent palatal torus. Metal (cast cobalt/chromium) bases will resist fracture but during function even they will flex slightly over a prominent palatal torus. The ultimate consequence is a fatigue fracture of the acrylic superstructure. No denture of conventional materials will provide satisfactory service. Polycarbonate may be tried but even with this the prognosis is poor; while polycarbonate has a high impact strength its other physical properties are little greater than conventional acrylic.[11] The material is a thermoplastic resin which cannot be formed by the dough process and must be manufactured by injection moulding with a corresponding increase in technical charges to account for the more complex equipment and the greater time involved.

Appearance

A complaint by the patient of poor appearance indicates that insufficient attention has been paid to this aspect at the try-in stage. However, an underlying worry about appearance should always be suspected when a patient's complaint, while not concerning appearance, persists despite correction of all other errors. Such patients consider it vanity to voice complaints about appearance and only sympathetic questioning by a knowledgeable clinician will elicit the appropriate responses.

Cleansing, aftercare and review

Instructions on denture cleansing will have been given at the end of the denture deilvery stage and the opportunity may now be taken of assessing the patient's reaction and the effect on oral hygiene. Disclosing agents are useful and provide a clear indication of lack of attention. The strictures once given against wearing complete dentures at night are no longer considered so valid, and can be relaxed when denture hygiene is optimal. The cleansing regimes that can be recommended are of two types, mechanical and chemical.

The simplest mechanical cleaner is a toothbrush, which can be used in association with either soap and water or with one of the proprietary denture cleansing pastes. Toothpastes can also be used and give a feeling of normality to the procedure. It is now known that the abrasives present in dentifrices do not cause noticeable damage to acrylic resin.[12] Special denture brushes can be bought and are probably better than conventional toothbrushes. They are larger and usually have design features which make them more efficient. Ideally plaque should be removed after every meal so that bacteria lack a plentiful carbohydrate substrate.

Elderly patients with arthritis may have problems when using denture toothbrushes, despite their large handles, just as they have when using conventional toothbrushes to clean natural teeth. It is unnecessary to make drastic alterations to the brush handle to make it more manipulable. Instead an immersion cleanser can be recommended. Cleansers may contain bleaches, detergents, oxidizing agents, hydrochloric acid and proteolytic enzymes, although the beneficial effect of the last additive is not yet certain. The best choice is probably one which contains hypochlorite, an ingredient with an excellent disinfectant and anti-plaque action. Alternatively, one containing a peroxide can be used, although the effervescent action does not appear to enhance the cleansing effect.

When using immersion cleansers, patients must be warned not to try to improve on the manufacturer's instructions. Bleaches and oxidizing agents will cause white discolouration of the denture-base resin if used for prolonged periods of time or at higher than recommended temperatures.[13] The advised temperatures are normally of the order of 30–40°C, and the denture should not remain immersed overnight in the active cleanser. Some cleansers containing hydrochloric acid are extremely effective in removing calcified deposits, but they should be used only with great care because they are equally effective in corroding any metal components. Warning must be given that when there is this risk hydrochloric acid cleansers should not be used.

A recent development in the field of denture cleansing is a small ultrasonic cleaner designed for this purpose.[14] It appears to be effective in its action and it seems ideal for any patient experiencing difficulty with normal routines. Best effect is probably achieved by using it in conjunction with a conventional chemical cleanser.

Aftercare for complete dentures is primarily directed to the removal of plaque and stain, and while patients are probably more concerned that stains are kept under control the dentist is more concerned to prevent candidal and similar infections. Both ends can be achieved with the relatively simple methods outlined above. Aftercare is more complex when a complete overdenture has been constructed. Here there is also the need to prevent caries of the abutments and aftercare must include some form of anti-caries therapy. Patients have to be encouraged to brush the abutments and reminded that a root abutment is in a particularly caries-prone site. Fluoride therapy is advisable. Patients can be recommended the use of fluoride mouth-rinses (0.05% fluoride) daily or they can be shown how to use acidulated phosphate fluoride gels (a drop placed inside the denture, over the abutments, at weekly intervals).

Regimes such as these require a high degree of cooperation from the patient, a quality which is in short supply among the elderly. Professional review by a hygienist is then a useful adjunct. Cleansing routines can be demonstrated, and their use reinforced at intervals of 2–3 months for the first year. As a further aid for overdenture wearers, fluoride varnishes can be applied. At later reviews the presence of caries can be detected at an early stage by use of microbiological tests developed for in-surgery use,[15] or by the application of stains to reveal dentine caries.[16]

With the review stage completed, patients are often allowed to determine their own time for recall, and it is often a long time before they consider it necessary. Cancer of the mouth is a very serious disease. Although its incidence is only 2% of all cancers, the 5-year survival rate for all except cancer of the lip is only 30–40%[17] and treatment is often severely mutilating. In England and Wales there are about 4000 cases of cancer of the mouth each year and 2000 deaths from this cause,[18] a statistic which reinforces the poor prognosis. When tumours are detected at a late stage, any surgery is especially mutilating, often involves block dissection of the neck tissues and is essentially palliative. The dentist is in an ideal situation to identify such lesions at

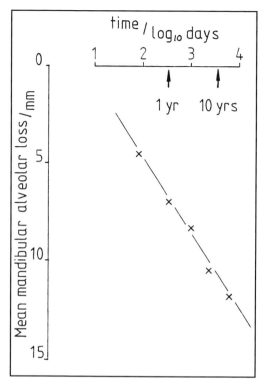

Fig. 8.5 Plot of mean mandibular vertical bone loss after extraction against log time. (Results adapted from: Tallgren, A. The continuing reduction of the residual alveolar ridge in complete denture wearers: a mixed-longitudinal study covering 25 years. *J Prosthet Dent* **27**:120–132, 1972.)

is most pronounced in the mandible and by plotting resorption against log time it can be shown that bone loss is progressive and that no denture can be considered permanent (Fig. 8.5). Naturally, more frequent review should be given to patients who have recently had extractions, who have a history of rapid resorption or who have been shown to adapt poorly to change.

The plot of resorption against log time also allows us to anticipate the amount of resorption to be expected in the case of an immediate complete denture. If we permit 2 mm of mandibular bone loss to be the maximum before modification is needed, either by temporary or permanent reline, then in the case of the average patient provision must be made for review of immediates at intervals of 1 month, 3 months and 1 year. At the last of these visits the dentures can be replaced by others which will last 2–3 years. If during the review period there is evidence that resorption is faster or slower than average, the frequency of review can be altered.

an early stage and initiate prompt referral and treatment. A good case can be made for recall and examination of elderly denture wearers at 1 year intervals when an inspection of the denture for deteriorating fit will not have the worrying implications that other monitoring procedures might have.

Apart from review for detection of pathology, the review of a denture cannot be allocated to set time intervals. Loss of retention results from resorption of alveolar bone, which process is itself continuous, the rate varying with individuals and the effect being noticeable soon after denture provision.[19] Alveolar resorption

References

1. Wilding, R.J.C. and Owen, C.P. The prevalence of temporomandibular joint dysfunction in edentulous non-denture wearing individuals. *J Oral Rehabil* **14**:175–182, 1987.
2. Devlin, H. and Watts, D.C. Acrylic "allergy". *Br Dent J* **157**:272–275, 1984.
3. Kazanji, M.N.M. and Watkinson, A.C. Influence of thickness, boxing and storage on the softness of resilient denture lining materials. *J Prosthet Dent* **59**:677–680, 1988.
4. Scott, J. Structure and function in aging human salivary glands. *Gerodontology* **5**:149–158, 1986.
5. McCartney, J.W. Flange adaptation discrepancy, palatal base distortion and

induced malocclusion caused by processing acrylic resin maxillary complete dentures. *J Prosthet Dent* **52**:545–553, 1984.

6. Langer, A. Chemopsychotherapy and its role in prosthodontic failures in elderly patients. *J Prosthet Dent* **52**:14–19, 1984.

7. Conny, D.J. and Tedesco, L.A. The gagging problem in prosthodontic treatment, Part II: patient mangement. *J Prosthet Dent* **49**:757–761, 1983.

8. Hoad-Reddick, G. Gagging: a chairside approach to control. *Br Dent J* **161**:174–176, 1986.

9. Petrovic, A. Speech sound distortions caused by changes in complete denture wearers. *J Oral Rehabil* **12**:69–79, 1985.

10. Hammond, R.J. and Beder, O.E. Increased vertical dimension and speech articulation errors. *J Prosthet Dent* **52**:401–406, 1984.

11. Stafford, G.D. and Smith, D.C. Polycarbonate: a preliminary report on the use of polycarbonate as a denture base material. *Dent Pract* **17**:217–223, 1967.

12. Murray, I.D., McCabe, J.F. and Storer, R. Abrasivity of denture cleansing pastes in vitro and in situ. *Br Dent J* **161**:137–141, 1986.

13. Arab, J., Newton, J.P. and Lloyd, C.H. The importance of water temperature on denture cleaning procedures. *J Dent* **16**:277–281, 1988.

14. Lees, A. A sound way to clean dentures. *Dent Pract.* **28**(7):19, 1990.

15. Stecksen-Blicks, C. Salivary counts of lactobacilli and *Streptococcus mutans* in caries prediction. *Scand J Dent Res* **93**:204–212, 1985.

16. Kidd, E.A.M., Joyston-Bechal, S., Smith, M.M., Allan, R., Howe, L. and Smith, S.R. The use of a caries detector dye in cavity preparation. *Br Dent J* **167**:132–134, 1989.

17. Smith, C.J. Oral cancer and precancer: background, epidemiology and aetiology. *Br Dent J* **167**:377–383, 1989.

18. Binnie, W.H., Cawson, R.A., Hill, G.B. and Soaper, A.E. Oral cancer in England and Wales: A national study of morbidity, mortality, curability and related factors. London: HMSO, 1972.

19. Berg, E. A 2-year follow-up study of patient satisfaction with complete new dentures. *J Dent* **16**:160–165, 1988.

Duplication and Copying Procedures

A patient's previous denture contains a great deal of information, especially if it has given many years of good service. Some of the available information can be used to aid construction of special trays without the need for primary impressions. Apart from the convenience of permitting this stage to be done by ancillary personnel, the technique is invaluable if the residual ridges are of a size or shape for which it would be difficult to obtain well fitting stock trays.

As a preliminary measure, additions are made in Greenstick composition to the periphery of the old denture in any place where it is judged to be underextended. A suitable amount of laboratory silicone putty is then mixed and an impression taken of the fitting surface. The bulk of the putty is moulded to form a conventionally shaped base (Fig. I.1). After the putty has set the denture is removed and returned to the patient. The "land" is trimmed with a scalpel to give the technician access to the periphery (Fig. I.2) and a special tray made on the silicone model to the clinician's prescription.

When it is desired to copy more of the desirable characteristics of the old denture a replica of it can be made in wax and autopolymerizing acrylic. Alginate is used as an investment material, being cheap and having handling properties familiar to the clinician. The most convenient duplicating flask is a soap dish,

selecting one with stops which precisely control the degree of closure (Fig. I.3). Avoid soap dishes made of polystyrene which are damaged by acrylic monomer.

The fitting surface of one of the pair of

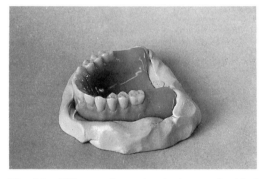

Fig. I.1 Fitting surface of a denture embedded in silicone putty.

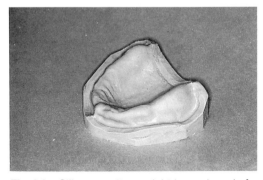

Fig. I.2 Silicone putty model trimmed ready for making special tray.

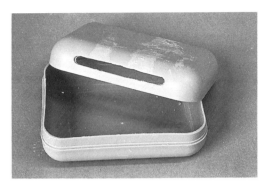

Fig. I.3 Suitable soap dish for denture copying. The slot aids escape of investment materials.

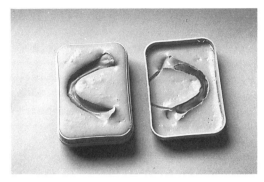

Fig. I.4 Impressions of the teeth filled with melted wax.

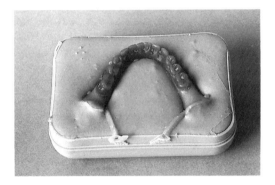

Fig. I.5 Denture replica after opening the dish.

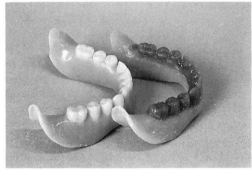

Fig. I.6 A comparison of the original denture and the trimmed replica.

selected dentures is first invested in alginate of normal consistency in the lower half of the dish, taking care to fill the fitting surface of the denture completely. When the first mix of alginate has set the opposite half of the dish is filled with a fluid mix of alginate and the first half inverted into it, allowing excess alginate to flow from a previously cut escape slot. When the second mix of alginate has set, the halves of the dish are separated and the denture removed and returned to the patient.

Pink wax is melted in a small galley pot and poured into the "tooth" side of the mould until the impressions of the teeth are filled (Fig. I.4). A mix of pink autopolymerizing acrylic is made and the remainder of the "tooth" side mould filled along with the mould of the "fitting" side. The dish is closed again, excess acrylic flowing to the exterior through the escape slot via shallow channels. After the acrylic has set the dish is opened (Fig. I.5) and the replica removed and trimmed (Fig. I.6). Simultaneous with the production of this replica a replica of the other denture is made, utilizing the times which would otherwise be wasted in waiting for materials to set.

If the occlusal surfaces of the original dentures are well marked and the cusps identifiable it is often possible to locate the occlusal surfaces of the two replicas together in the intercuspal position. If not an occlusal record must be made. The replicas are then sent to the technician with instructions to mount on an articulator and replace the wax teeth one by one with new teeth of a selected shade. At the following visit a try-in is made, and if the patient is satisfied with the appearance, closed-mouth impressions are made in the replicas using a fluid silicone, having removed any undercuts from the bases. While this serves to eliminate any remaining errors in the registration, the two layers of silicone rubber will also make a small increase in the face height. Fortunately, small increases of this order are usually desirable to compensate for alveolar resorption. The work is returned to the technician, models cast and the try-ins processed as normal.

For those occasions when an increase in face height is to be made, greater than that expected to result from the extra thickness of impression material, the replicas are tried in the patient's mouth before the teeth are added, immediately after they have been made and trimmed. At this preliminary try-in any alterations to the face height can be made by wax additions to the occlusal surfaces before sending it to the technician for further work as above.

By this technique the occlusal and polished surfaces of the old denture are reproduced and the period of adjustment to a new denture made easier—only the fitting surface is changed to any considerable extent. The technique is invaluable when dealing with an elderly person for whom a prolonged period of adaptation to new dentures is to be expected. The elderly are also grateful to find the number of clinical visits reduced to a

minimum. It is also useful as a technique for making a spare denture for any patient who is concerned to think that fracture or loss will result in having to live for a time without dentures.

The great advantage of making the template with an acrylic base and wax superstructure lies in the different needs which the composite structure satisfies. Wax is easily cut and removed by the technician when adding teeth to the replica, while the acrylic base is resistant to distortion during clinical procedures and serves as an adequately strong backing for the impression.

A third way in which a copying process can simplify clinical procedures also involves making a replica as above. In this case the replicas are used as registration blocks, the wax teeth serving as rims to which additions and changes can be made to modify the final tooth prescription. Inevitably, registration blocks manufactured in this way are a poor fit, being made to a ridge form which existed when the original dentures were first made. To eliminate inaccuracy, closed mouth impressions are made in the registration blocks using silicone rubber, before final adjustments are made and the horizontal jaw relations established. Models are cast to the bases by the technician who mounts them on an articulator and produces a try-in with teeth of the clinician's choosing. The impression material is retained on the base of the try-in to ensure an accurate fit for the clinical stage. Silicone rubber is the imperative choice for the impression material; only a tough elastomeric impression material will resist the remaining technical and clinical procedures in a relatively undamaged form.

Appendix II

Permanent Reline Procedures

Resorption of alveolar bone is a continuous process and complete dentures, especially mandibular dentures, soon lose their accurate fit. Overall stability is only preserved for a while by the muscle control which develops with time. The useful life of a denture can be prolonged by relining the fitting surface, and it is to be expected that reline procedures are of most use in association with immediate dentures and during the first few years following loss of the teeth. Differences in resorption rates between the mandible and maxilla also ensure that mandibular dentures are relined far more frequently than maxillary.

Two problems tend to occur as a result of reline techniques. The first is an increase in face height as a consequence of the added thickness of the reline impression material. Usually this is acceptable and compensates for the loss of face height following on resorption. Unfortunately the loss of height due to resorption tends to occur at the expense of the mandible and if both dentures are to be relined, unless great care is taken to ensure that no increase in thickness of the maxillary denture base takes place, there will be a lowering of the occlusal plane and an objectionable change in appearance.

The other problem is particularly liable to occur when the mandible is atrophic, namely a problem in correctly locating the denture, made worse by the intervening layer of impression material which diminishes the operator's tactile sense. Because small discrepancies are almost inevitable, it is best to complete a reline procedure by a check record and readjustment of the occlusal surfaces.

Reline procedures start with removing any undercuts from the fitting surfaces, otherwise it will prove impossible to remove the denture from the model that will be cast onto it. Where an initial underextension is diagnosed any small additions are made to the periphery in an appropriate material. Reline impressions are best made in silicone rubber. Skilled practitioners can utilize silicones of different viscosities in order to vary the degree to which an increase in the face height is made. Where no increase is to be made, and always in the case of a maxillary denture, a fluid silicone is best. Also in the case of maxillary dentures, holes are cut through the palatal surface to allow flow of the impression material and seating of the maxillary denture in close contact with the mucoperiosteum.

With the opposing denture in place, the denture to be relined is inserted, positioned as accurately as possible, and the patient asked to close in the retruded contact position. Ensure that impression material extrudes from the entire periph-

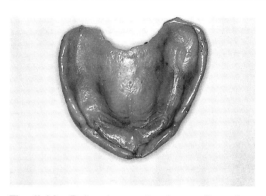

Fig. II.1A Reline impression in maxillary denture showing the fitting surface of a completed impression.

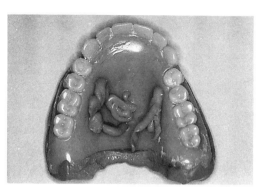

Fig. II.1B Polished surface of denture with extrusion of excess impression material through relief holes in the palate.

ery and continue as for making a normal impression (Figs II.1A and II.1B.). When increases in face height are proposed the thickness of the set impression material can be estimated by penetration with a sharp probe and the procedure repeated until the thickness is satisfactory.

Permanent relines are often made of autopolymerizing acrylic resin. While the physical properties are not ideal, it is justifiable on the grounds of ease of technique and the fact that if an immediate denture is being relined (as is often the case) it will be expected to last a relatively short period of time before a more permanent replacement will be made. If normal heat-cured resin is requested, a long cure at 70°C is advisable to prevent distortion of the original base by stress relief.

When after a reline there is no improvement in retention, even after a check record has eliminated occlusal faults, suspect a misdiagnosis. Any clinician contemplating a permanent reline should make certain that the problem to be corrected is one of lack of retention or instability due to resorption. Where it is instability due to interference with muscle action, or even lack of interocclusal space, relining the denture will only make the problem worse.

Appendix III

Use of an Adjustable Articulator

The Dentatus ARL or ARH is a popular, simple, non-Arcon, adjustable articulator which is satisfactory for complete denture prosthodontics. It has a reference plane which corresponds to the Frankfort plane, from the lower border of the left orbit, through the heads of the condyles. The simplified technique described here makes some allowance for the decreased stability of the mandibular registration block in an edentulous subject and by spreading the work over two visits avoids overstressing elderly patients.

Clinical procedures are as normal up to the jaw registration, at which stage the face bow is used to transfer the maxillo-mandibular relations to the articulator. When the registration blocks have been adjusted and the correct face height established, the blocks are removed from the patient's mouth and the bite fork firmly embedded in the buccal surface of the upper rim. Ensure that the rod connecting the fork to the facebow emerges from the mouth on the right hand side and that the bite fork index ring is in the midline (Fig. III.1).

With a pencil, mark on the patient's face the estimated positions of the condyles, 1 cm in front of the tragus of the ear, on a line joining the tragus with the commissure of the eye. Replace both blocks in the patient's mouth and locate

them together in the retruded contact position. Take the facebow and attach it loosely to the bite fork by means of the corresponding slip joint. While the DSA holds the cup ends of the bow over the marked condyle heads, adjust the facebow cursors until the readings are equal. Take the infra-orbital pointer, slide it through the (patient's) left hand slip joint and bring the tip into contact with the left infra-orbital margin at the lowest point (Fig. III.2.). Tighten all the slip joints, adjust both cursors to zero and remove the entire assembly from the patient in one piece.

In the laboratory the assembly is mounted on the articulator via the cups on the facebow, again having equalized the cursors. The height of the adjustment

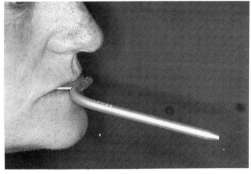

Fig. III.1 Bite fork embedded in the rim of a registration block. The index mark is in the midline.

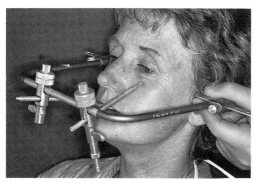

Fig. III.2 Face bow in position on the patient, supported anteriorly by bite fork and posteriorly by DSA.

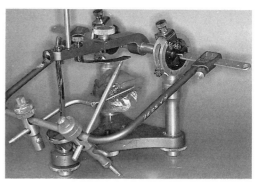

Fig. III.3 Face bow and models mounted on the articulator with the infra-orbital pointer in contact with the infra-orbital plate.

screw on the bow is altered to bring the infra-orbital pointer into contact with the infra-orbital plane guide on the articulator (Fig. III.3.) The working models are mounted in turn in the blocks and plastered to their respective arms of the articulator. A balanced articulation is set up with an incisal guidance angle of 10° and after adjusting the condyle angles to an initial setting of 40°.

If the try-in is satisfactory a recording is made of the sagittal condylar angle using a silicone putty registration of the Christiansen phenomenon. After the patient has practised closing into a protruded mandibular contact position about 5–6 mm in front of the retruded contact position (edge-to-edge is often easier to describe to the patient), a protrusive record in silicone putty is made (the alternative—wax—is more susceptible to distortion). Placing the try-in back on the articulator, the occlusal surfaces of the teeth are related to each other by means of the protrusive record. The condylar guidance angles are altered in turn until even contact occurs in the record, when

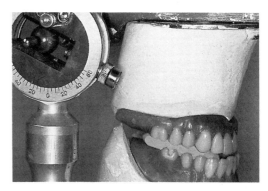

Fig. III.4 Teeth related via a protrusive record. With the condylar guidance set at 20° the maxillary canine teeth are displaced from the record. If the condylar guidance angle were too great, a similar space would appear posteriorly. At an intermediate setting even contact occurs.

the adjustment is locked (Fig. III.4). An average Bennett shift is incorporated by rotating the condylar pillars inwards 15°.

Adjustments are now made to the angulations of the teeth to allow a new balanced articulation to be established. When complete, the try-in is invested, processed and finished.

Index